FLU

Other books by Randall Neustaedter

The Vaccine Guide:
Risks and Benefits for Children and Adults

Child Health Guide:
Holistic Pediatrics for Parents

FLU

Alternative Treatments and Prevention

**Proven Strategies to Protect
Yourself and Your Family**

Randall Neustaedter, OMD

North Atlantic Books
Berkeley, California

Published by
North Atlantic Books
P.O. Box 12327
Berkeley, California 94712

ISBN 1-55643-568-1
Library of Congress Catalogue Card Number 2004026993

Cover and book design by Paula Morrison
Printed in the United States of America
Distributed to the book trade by Publishers Group West

Flu: Alternative Treatments and Prevention is sponsored by the Society for the Study of Native Arts and Sciences, a nonprofit educational corporation whose goals are to develop an educational and crosscultural perspective linking various scientific, social, and artistic fields; to nurture a holistic view of arts, sciences, humanities, and healing; and to publish and distribute literature on the relationship of mind, body, and nature.

Disclaimer: The following information is intended for general information purposes only. Individuals should always see their health care provider before administering any suggestions made in this book. Any application of the material set forth in the following pages is at the reader's discretion and is his or her sole responsibility.

1 2 3 4 5 6 7 8 9 DATA 10 09 08 07 06 05

Contents

Preface

Every winter brings rain, snow, and the flu. Sometimes the flu season is mild; in other years it causes widespread debilitating illness, and periodically it rages with a force that proves devastating. The public feels helpless confronting another flu season, hoping for the best. Seniors and residents of nursing homes dread the possibility of an illness that can easily progress to pneumonia and dire consequences. Vaccination against the flu has been hailed as the primary and best preventive, but the shortage of flu vaccine in 2004 and the controversies surrounding the lack of effectiveness of vaccination have led many people to seek alternatives.

Fortunately, you can prepare for the flu season with effective prevention strategies. If the flu does strike, you can also treat the symptoms with safe alternative methods. This book will guide you to the most effective alternative strategies for managing the flu with appropriate professional care and treatment you can do yourself at home.

There is a great deal of fear of the flu generated by the media. Most of this fear stems from the inability of conventional medicine to treat the flu, or other viral illnesses, with any degree of success. Alternative medical practices, by contrast, have accumulated a record of consistently effective treatments for the flu that also prevent complications. Homeopathy is especially successful at managing flu symptoms.

The first part of this book tells the history of flu, and describes flu symptoms and complications. There's also a discussion of flu vaccines and the vaccine shortage. Part II describes the alternative medical approaches you can use to treat the flu, and important measures you can adopt to build a strong immune system that will help you avoid the flu and its complications. In Part III you will learn methods for flu prevention and treatment in children. And Part IV will guide you to the best ways to increase immunity, treat the flu, and prevent the serious complications of the flu for adults and seniors. No matter what your state of health or your risk for complications, you need to know the best possible natural, alternative methods for handling the threat and dangers of this harrowing illness.

Part I

Flu and the Vaccine
The Flu
Short history of influenza

The word *influenza* is Italian for *influence,* as in the astral or occult influence of a visitation or outbreak that affects many people at the same time. First used in 1504, the word signified any disease epidemic. In a severe flu outbreak of 1743 the word influenza was applied to the epidemic that began in Italy and spread throughout Europe. Since then influenza, shortened to flu, means a serious infectious disease characterized by muscle and joint aching, prostration, and respiratory congestion with fever and headache. We often hear the word flu also loosely applied to any type of contagious respiratory or digestive infection or disturbance, as in the "stomach flu."

It was not until 1931 that an influenza virus was identified in pigs, and finally in 1933 a human influenza virus was discovered by three British researchers: Smith, Andrewes, and Laidlaw. Both of these viruses were closely related to the

Spanish flu virus of 1918. During the time of the 1918 flu pandemic, however, the suspected culprit was a bacterium named *Hemophilus influenza*. Viruses had not yet been discovered.

Although most people consider the flu simply an annoyance, and possibly a danger to seniors in poor health, influenza has been responsible for repeated, devastating worldwide pandemics capable of bringing entire nations to their knees. It is hard for us to imagine today, but in 1918 the entire world was in the clutches of a deadly flu virus. The 1918 flu still remains the greatest plague the world has ever seen.

Hippocrates recorded an epidemic of a flu-like infection in 412 B.C. that wiped out the Athenian army. The sixteenth century saw two flu pandemics that spread throughout Europe. The first, in 1510, infected nearly the entire population of Europe, but claimed few lives. The second, in 1580, devastated cities and spread through the whole of Western Europe. The city of Rome, for example, had 9,000 fatalities. At least three pandemics of flu spread throughout Europe in the seventeenth century. In the past 200 years eight great flu pandemics seized the world prior to the devastation wrought by the 1918 flu. During a period of fourteen months beginning in the spring of 1918, half of the entire world's population was infected with the

THE SPREAD OF FLU

Endemic: occurring in a particular place: within a specific area, region, or locale. Example: The bird flu was endemic to Thailand.

Epidemic: fast-spreading: an outbreak that spreads more quickly and more extensively among a group of people than would normally be expected. Example: Officials predict a widespread winter flu epidemic this year.

Pandemic: having widespread effect: existing in the form of a widespread epidemic that affects people in many different countries. Example: The 1918 flu pandemic killed an estimated 40 million people worldwide.

influenza virus, and nearly 40 million people died. Every country in the world was affected, no matter how remote, and this occurred in an era before air travel and a global community existed. Victims who died during the 1918 flu were typically healthy young adults. Among the 20-to-40-year-old age group, the fatality rate from the 1918 flu was 50 percent. The virus of 1918 was so effective at killing its host that within a short period of time it rendered itself extinct. People were either immune to the virus or dead. Since that time several other lesser pandemics have occurred across the globe, but health officials anxiously await the next deadly flu pandemic, which they predict as inevitable. When it occurs, experts foresee millions of deaths, hospitals quickly flooded with cases of pneumonia, and every health care system in the world overwhelmed by the volume of flu victims.

Viral attack

The influenza virus is a bit of protein, a membrane surrounding eight genes. It is a simple but sophisticated killing machine with a mission to multiply. The flu virus takes the shape of a sphere with spikes protruding from its surface. The spikes are primarily invaders that attach to epithelial cells on the surface of mucous membranes in the airways of animals. The spikes, composed of a glycoprotein called hemagglutinin, bind to a cell, and hold the virus tightly to the cell's wall while the virus creates a hole in the cell. Then the virus simply slips through this hole and enters the cell. Once the influenza virus hides inside the cell, the body's immune system cannot find it and destroy it. The virus then has all the time it needs to do its work. This sneak attack is a special trick of the influenza virus, and accounts for its great success.

Researchers have analyzed the 1918 flu virus taken from autopsy specimens during that pandemic to discover what made it such an effective killer. They synthesized the gene for the hemagglutinin spike and used it to produce the viral protein and analyze it. It is the peculiar structure of the hemagglutinin spike on the membrane of the 1918 virus that accounted for its deadly effect. The hemagglutinin that previously could only bind to bird cells evolved to a highly unusual form that could easily spread to humans. This ability to effectively bind to human cells, coupled with the novel protein structure that the immune system of humans could not recognize or defeat, made the 1918 virus an especially destructive force (Gamblin, 2004).

The job of the influenza virus is to take control in the cell's nucleus, issuing commands to build more viral proteins. The virus copies its genes using the genetic material of human cells, combines them with the viral proteins produced by the cell, and forms new viral particles. About ten hours after initial contact with the cell membrane, the virus has reproduced at an astonishing rate. Between 100,000 and 1 million new viruses have been produced. Then the cell explodes and dies. Mutations also occur at an astonishing rate, creating an elusive enemy that can readily adapt to new terrain. Only 1 percent of the new viruses will survive as a result of these random mutations. That leaves 1,000 to 10,000 efficient invaders to quickly attack other epithelial cells. Within a very short time, the entire epithelial surface of the throat or bronchial airway becomes a devastated wasteland. Then the body reacts, mobilizing an immune response.

An army of white blood cells floods the area of infection, along with specific antibodies against the new viral proteins and cytokines that stimulate inflammation. It is the cytokines produced by white blood cells that cause most of the symptoms of flu. These protein messengers cause the body to raise its temperature and are responsible for the headache, muscle aches, and increased mucus production characteristic of the flu. The dryness and rawness of mucous membranes is accomplished by the virus firestorm that has denuded vast areas of the protective layer of the respiratory tract. The most dangerous symptoms, however, occur in the lungs.

Particularly effective flu viruses quickly march into the lungs and begin their slash-and-burn process in the epithelial cells that line the alveoli, the tiny air sacs at the end of the respiratory tree where oxygen is exchanged. Then the immune system goes on the attack, flooding the area with white cells, antibodies, and cytokines. An inflammatory defense ensues with accumulation of fluid, blood, and debris from the battle. The alveoli fill with this fluid, replacing the air, and large areas of lung become dense and damaged. The result is pneumonia. If it is widespread, lack of oxygen becomes a serious problem, fluid cannot be pumped out of the lungs fast enough, and the flu victim drowns, or the heart works so hard trying to accomplish this drainage that congestive heart failure occurs.

Flu virus by the numbers

Classification of flu viruses is a complicated business. Here is a crash course. The flu viruses are named and numbered. The 1918 Spanish flu was an H1N1 A flu virus. Influenza viruses come in three varieties—A, B, and C—each with different nucleoproteins (NP) encoded by the NP gene. A viruses are more virulent and responsible for the major flu epidemics. B viruses typically cause milder symptoms and more sporadic disease spread. C viruses seldom cause symptoms. Flu vaccines contain two A viruses and a B virus.

Two types of proteins (hemagglutinin and neuraminidase) sit in the outer membrane of the virus, and serve to identify the virus in the H and N coding system. The HA gene encodes the hemagglutinin protein responsible for the spikes that bind to cell membranes. Three types of hemagglutinin affect humans: H1, H2, and H3. Nine others have been identified that affect animals. The NA gene encodes the neuraminidase protein, which is the part of the viral membrane that protects it from the cell's defenses.

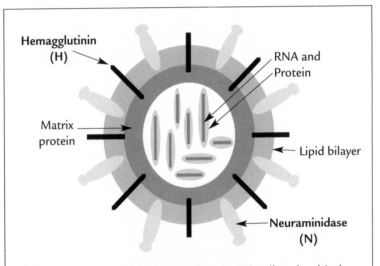

Influenza A virus with its hemagglutinin (H) spikes that bind to target cells in the body and neuraminidase (N) spikes that protect the virus from the body's defenses.

There are two—N1 and N2. That's about it. The most worrisome flu viruses currently in circulation are different strains of the H3N2 line, the A/Panama, A/Fujian, and A/Wellington, each named for the place where it was first discovered. Bird flu is an H5 virus, H5N1.

Virologists are certain that another great flu pandemic will occur in the next ten years, probably arising in China where contact between birds and humans is common and

HUMAN FLU VIRUS CLASSIFICATION

Virus type		hemagglutinin	neuraminidase
A	Epidemics	H1	N1
		H2	N2
		H3	
B	Mild symptoms		
C	No symptoms		

frequent in open-air street markets (Li, 2004). All of the "modern"-era flu pandemics (1957, 1968, 1976) originated in China. Scientists insist that every flu pandemic in history has been spread from animals to humans. The Spanish flu of 1918 was probably transmitted to humans by pigs. Other flu viruses have made the species jump from birds. In recent years, deadly bird flu viruses of the H5N1 variety have also been transmitted to humans, most recently in Southeast Asia, where scores of deaths resulted.

Public health experts predict that the random mutations in bird flu viruses will inevitably create an efficient killer once again. Typically, infection by a flu virus will leave the sufferer immune to that strain, but viruses have a remarkable ability to mutate, creating new strains that the human host's immune system will not recognize. This has

THE FLU VIRUSES	
1918 Spanish flu	A/H1N1
1957 Asian flu	A/H2N2
1968 Hong Kong flu	A/H3N2
1976 Swine flu	A/H1N1
2003 Fujian flu	A/H3N2
2004 Bird flu	A/H5N1

enabled the elusive flu virus to continue its march through human history. However, even new strains of viruses will be similar enough to previously encountered versions so that the immune system will recognize and defeat the new invader (Davies, 1989). It is the completely different virus, never previously encountered, that proves devastating. An animal such as a bird or rodent harbors a virus, passes this virus to humans, and the new encounter destroys the host before the immune system can mount an adequate response. Viruses mutate at an enormously high rate. It takes only one random mutation to develop a bird virus that fits a perfect niche, a virus that is able to easily bind to human cells while evading the immune system and still be easily transmitted between humans. Once that rare set of circumstances occurs, researchers say, a pandemic is likely (Li, 2004). In 1918 the H1 virus was novel enough to take hold in the human body with remarkable tenacity. In 1957 it was the new H2 virus, or Asian flu, that caused the pandemic, and in 1968 the H3, or Hong Kong strain. Each of these viruses came from birds. That is why scientists and public health officials worry so much about new bird viruses today. Recently, the H5N1 avian virus has been causing the entire world to shake with trepidation.

DEADLY ENCOUNTERS

At the end of August 2004, an 11-year-old girl was helping her aunt to destroy some dead chickens in their remote village in northern Thailand. On September 2, 2004, she became sick and was hospitalized. The girl's 26-year-old mother, Pranee, was working in Bangkok at the time. She returned home to care for her sick daughter in the hospital, but on September 12 the girl died. Pranee returned to Bangkok after her daughter's death, but she too was taken ill, and within a few days, on September 20, she also died of an H5 bird flu virus apparently contracted from her daughter. This tragic family drama would be heart-rending enough. What makes it especially terrifying is the ability of the bird flu virus to spread from person to person, a route of transmission that health officials fear could spark another flu pandemic. The aunt, her 3-year-old son, and nine other people in the region also contracted the H5 virus. A 13-year-old also died. The avian flu epidemic has been declared "a crisis of global proportions."

Avian flu control methods extend across Asia and the entire world, routinely prompting the slaughter of entire flocks of birds that may be infected. In 1997 public health officials in Hong Kong decided to kill every bird within its borders. Despite these preventive measures, officials still worry about the spread of disease. Avian flu viruses can persist in bird feces for days or weeks after birds have been slaughtered. Truck tires or boots of clean-up crews can spread the disease, making control measures difficult. Mammals contract the disease, increasing the number of possible hosts. During the fall of 2004, tigers at a zoo in Thailand spread the disease from cat to cat, killing twenty of the valuable animals. The ability of the virus to spread between mammals or between people has public health officials extremely worried.

EAGLES AT THE AIRPORT

On October 17, 2004, a Thai man traveled on an EVA Airways flight from Bangkok to Vienna and caught a connecting flight to Belgium. At a routine drug check at the airport in Brussels, customs officers found two small, crested hawk eagles still alive in plastic tubes in the man's carry-on bags. Transporting birds from Thailand is illegal, and the man had no permits for importing the endangered eagle species. Since Belgian law has no provisions for detaining smugglers, authorities released the man, but seized the birds, which were barely alive. The eagles proved to have the H5N1 virus, and they were killed, along with 200 parrots that had been exposed to the infected eagles while awaiting shipment to a pet shop. Four hundred other smaller birds were exposed but transported out of the airport before the eagles were tested. The vet who killed the eagles developed an eye infection, a typical symptom of bird flu virus in humans. The man who smuggled the birds surrendered to Belgian authorities after a nationwide public appeal. He was treated preventively for the flu. This narrow escape shows how easily a localized epidemic could spread from Asia to the Western world. If that bird flu virus happened to be aggressive, then exposure of travelers in a plane compartment or an airport could spark a conflagration.

Symptoms

You've probably had the flu sometime in the past and know how it feels from personal experience. In case you have forgotten the feeling, here are the typical symptoms. A day or two after exposure to someone with the flu, you feel a bit out of sorts for a day. Then the next day or that night, you are knocked flat with unmistakable muscle aching, chills, a dreadful headache, and dry cough. You languish in bed, taking painkillers for the headache, drinking fluids, and waiting for the ordeal to end. In a few days it does. You have lost a few pounds and five days of work. You feel weak for another four days, then after ten to fourteen days back to normal. If you are lucky. Some people develop pneumonia, the most common complication of the flu. Since the pneumonia is usually viral, antibiotics are useless. Sometimes people will recover from the flu and then another high fever develops with typical pneumonia symptoms of coughing, chest tightness, difficulty breathing, and weakness. This secondary infection is often bacterial. Deaths typically occur as a result of pneumonia.

IT'S JUST THE FLU—HOW BAD CAN IT GET?

Sarah woke at 6:00 a.m. on Tuesday morning with a

scratchy sore throat. She prepared her children's lunches, and then put a pot of oatmeal on for their breakfast. Her husband had left earlier that morning for a short business trip. By the time Karen dropped the children off at school, she could feel the telltale signs of a fever, the light head, the faint flush of a cold sweat, and a tight, nagging ache in her shoulders. I don't have time for this today, she thought. By the time she arrived at her own office, she began to wonder if she would make it through the day. Her vision was swimming and a dull pounding had begun in her temples. Fortunately, she kept a bottle of aspirin in her desk, but by the time her supervisor stopped in to say hello at ten, her slumped posture and glazed eyes prompted him to send her home. He could ill afford to have the entire office infected.

She arrived home at noon, barely able to climb the stairs to her bed. Perhaps a short nap would revive her. As she climbed into bed, she ignored her clothing, grateful for the warmth of the comforter that might alleviate the shaking chills that overtook her. Despite the pounding pressure in her head, she eventually fell asleep. By the time the children came home from school, she could barely control the coughing fits that would rack her body, each paroxysm of cough causing a searing pain through her chest. And the fullness in her chest, the copious secretion of mucus coughed from her lungs, did worry her when she had a few moments of coherent thought.

Her oldest daughter, Josie, was capable enough to fix dinner for the younger children and get them to bed. Josie asked her mother if she should contact the family doctor. "I'll go see him tomorrow," Sarah assured her daughter.

That night Karen slept fitfully between coughing spells. A nosebleed proved peculiarly difficult to stop. Her breathing came in gasps with bands of steel binding her chest and a burning rawness in her air passages. At 11:00 she woke from a frightening dream of swimming against a current, unable to keep her head above the waves. She reached for the light, alarmed at all the wetness. The pillows and bedclothes were soaked and red. Horrified and confused, she could not remember where she was or what to do. Without strength or will, getting herself out of bed was not even a consideration.

Time of death, 2:00 a.m., October 8, 1918.

During the month of October 1918 in America, 195,000 people died of the flu, many of them within eighteen hours of disease onset. The worldwide flu pandemic claimed an estimated 40 million lives. No one knows exactly why that particular virus was so deadly, but the gruesome descriptions of cases rival any medical accounts of the Black plague, smallpox, or ebola virus. Physicians described patients who literally bled to death before their eyes in 1918, spurting blood from nosebleeds, oozing blood from the eyes or ears, and hemorrhaging from the lungs, intestines, and uterus. Pneumonia usually began within a day or two after exposure, followed by high fever and convulsions. The lungs were literally destroyed and laid waste by the flu bug. The skin turned purple prior to death from lack of oxygen in the bloodstream, a certain sign of impending doom. The total death toll from the flu in America in 1918–1919 was 675,000, a proportion of the population that in the current era would total 1,750,000. Despite these dire scenarios, homeopathic physicians had tremendous success in treating the 1918 flu and remarkably reduced fatalities compared to their conventional colleagues (see page 34).

Complications and deaths

Modern flu epidemics bear little resemblance to the horrors of the 1918 flu and other deadly pandemics. The popular media, including newspapers (*Los Angeles Times* Editorial, Oct. 19, 2004) and television shows (NBC's Today Show, Oct. 6, 2004) tell us that 36,000 flu deaths occur each year. This statistic comes from an article published in the *Journal of the American Medical Association* in 2003 that *estimated* flu deaths (Thompson, 2003). However, the official statistics from the Centers for Disease Control (CDC) cite the average total death rate from flu at about 1,000 per year during the period 1999–2002 (CDC, 2004a). Nonetheless, the *Washington Post* predicted 50,000 deaths from the flu in the 2004–05 flu season (Oct. 17, 2004, David Brown, staff writer). Perhaps Mark Twain spoke for others beside himself when he said, "The reports of my death are highly exaggerated."

The most frequent complication of flu is pneumonia, which occurs primarily in children under 2 and in seniors. Viral pneumonia can be a deadly force, killing within forty-eight hours of disease onset. Apparently, most pneumonias that occurred in the 1918 flu were viral. The influenza virus can disable and overwhelm the immune system. Most deaths occur from viral pneumonia because the body creates such a dramatic immune response to the virus that it floods the lungs with fluids in its attempt to attack the multiplying viruses. Secondary bacterial pneumonia takes longer to develop and can be treated more effectively. Bacterial pneumonia may occur because the virus specifically helps bacteria attach to lung tissue. Pneumonia should be suspected in anyone who has a painful, loose-sounding cough and difficult, labored breathing or rapid breathing.

DEATHS FROM FLU AND PNEUMONIA		
	Flu	Pneumonia
1999	1,665	62,065
2000	1,765	63,548
2001	257	61,777
2002	727	65,954

Guillain-Barré Syndrome is a rare complication of the flu characterized by an autoimmune response that causes damage to the sheaths of nerves, resulting in tingling, numbness, weakness, and eventual paralysis of the extremities. If it affects the muscles of respiration, the illness can end in suffocation.

Viral encephalitis occurs when the flu virus attacks the brain. Symptoms are extreme lethargy, confusion, and inability to waken from sleep.

Flu Vaccines
Choosing a virus

Each year teams of researchers make recommendations to vaccine manufacturers about the viruses that should be included in the next year's flu vaccine. Manufacturers need at least nine months lead time to produce the next year's vaccine supply. By January they must decide what vaccine to have ready by October.

Choosing the three viruses to include in the vaccine is educated guesswork. Scientists have discovered that migrating wild ducks and domestic pigs in Asia carry viruses that may appear in the following year's flu epidemics. These animals are slaughtered and the viruses they harbor are used to determine the strains of flu to use in the vaccine. The problem is that these predictions do not always prove to be accurate. There are years when the predominant flu virus is not contained in the vaccine. This occurred during the winter of 2003, when the predominant flu virus strain (A/Fujian H3N2) differed from the vaccine strain. The result was a vaccine with no effectiveness against influenza-like illnesses, according to a study conducted by the Centers for Disease Control (CDC, 2004).

Similar situations have occurred in other years as well. According to a CDC report on the 1994–1995 flu season, 87 percent of type A influenza virus samples from flu victims were not similar to the year's vaccine, and 76 percent of type B virus were not similar to the virus in that year's vaccine. During the 1992–1993 season, 84 percent of samples for the predominant type A virus were not similar to the virus in the vaccine. The flu vaccine for any particular year faces similar challenges. In the fall of 2004, the A/Wellington virus strain defied the vaccine manufacturers, who had included the previous year's A/Fujian virus strain in the vaccine. If a virus other than the ones contained in the vaccine takes hold in a population, then the flu vaccine will again have missed the mark that year.

Effectiveness

Most people assume that the flu vaccine will protect them from the flu, and flu vaccine is purported to be 70–90 percent effective when the viral strains match the circulating disease. But studies have not always confirmed the flu vaccine's effectiveness, especially in the groups most vulnerable to the complications of flu—children under 2 and seniors. A recommendation was made for the 2004–2005 flu season to vaccinate all children ages 6–24 months. This recommendation was not based on proven effectiveness of the vaccine in this age group, but because two studies showed that these young children had more hospitalizations from the flu than older children (see page 72). In an enthusiastic effort to protect these young children, the vaccine was rushed to the marketplace. A recent study from Japan, however, showed that the flu shot did not reduce the attack rate of influenza A infection in 6–24-month-old children. During the years 2000–2002, groups of children in this age range were designated to either receive the vaccine or act as controls with no flu vaccination. The two groups were observed from January to April in each of the three years. At the end of this time the attack rates of influenza in the two groups were nearly the same, and no protective advantage was found from the flu shot (Maeda, 2004).

The primary targeted group for flu vaccine is seniors, yet the vaccine has not proven especially protective for that population. The relative ineffectiveness of the flu vaccine in seniors is undoubtedly due to the diminishing immune response, particularly of T cells, as people age (Pawelec, 2003). According to the CDC, the effectiveness of flu vaccine in preventing illness among elderly people residing in nursing homes is 30–40 percent (CDC, 2001). Other studies have shown an even lower efficacy of 0–36 percent (averaging 21 percent). The CDC proudly notes that for those living outside of nursing homes, flu vaccine is 30–70 percent effective in preventing hospitalization for pneumonia and influenza. Yet the Department of Human and Health Services found that, with or without a flu shot, pneumonia and influenza hospitalization rates for the elderly are less than 1 percent during the influenza season.

Regardless of vaccination status, 99 percent of seniors recover from the flu without being hospitalized.

Adverse effects of the vaccine

According to the CDC, the most common side effects of the flu vaccine include fever, fatigue, muscle aches, and headache. The presence of formaldehyde and mercury preservatives has also fueled controversy over the safety of the vaccine.

However, the most significant and dreaded side effect of the flu vaccine is Guillain-Barré Syndrome (GBS), an autoimmune nervous system reaction characterized by unstable gait, loss of sensation, and loss of muscle control. In 1976 a mass flu vaccination program was mounted by the U.S. government. That campaign ended when vaccine recipients in Ohio developed GBS at a rate six times the normal incidence in non-recipients (Marks, 1980). Michigan and Minnesota reported similar increased rates of GBS in vaccinees (Safranek, 1991). More recently, an increased risk for GBS occurring in patients during the six weeks following vaccination was revealed in the 1992–1993 and the 1993–1994 flu seasons (Lasky, 1998).

Vaccine shortage

A total of 100 million doses of flu vaccine were produced for the 2004–2005 flu season. However, a major setback to flu vaccine dissemination occurred when the entire supply from one of the two companies producing vaccine was seized due to bacterial contamination at the manufacturing facility in Liverpool, England. This left the U.S. with only 55 million doses of vaccine and the need to ration those doses to seniors and small children—those who had the highest risk of complications. Most children and adults were left without the benefit of vaccine protection.

The vaccine shortage occurred because profits from flu vaccines are marginal and most companies had quit vaccine production. In the 1970s more than twelve companies made flu shots. In 2004 that number had dwindled to only two companies. Profits are limited because sales of vaccine depend upon demand, which is fueled by anxiety over this year's flu epidemic. If vaccine manufacturers do not generate sales, then their product must be discarded, because each year they create a new, current vaccine. In the 2000–2001 season, 8 million doses were discarded. In 2001–2002, another 10 million, and in 2002–2003, a total of 13 million doses went into the dumpster. That comes to a total of $50 million in unsold vaccine. In October 2004, the loss of 48 million doses of vaccine by Chiron amounted to a $91-million write-off, reducing the company's earnings by 36 cents a share. Following the closing of the Liverpool vaccine facility, Chiron came under federal investigation and was sued by the company's shareholders for making misleading statements about their ability to produce the vaccine.

A study published subsequent to the vaccine shortage crisis of 2004 showed that it may be possible to reduce the dose of the flu vaccine by one-fifth in young adults (age 18–40) and still stimulate antibody protection at levels assumed to be protective (Kenney, 2004). A second study evaluated a dose one-third the size of the standard vaccine (Belshe, 2004). The two studies showed similar or greater levels of protective antibody in the group that received the lowered dose, compared to the group that received the full dose of vaccine. The reduced-dose technique requires an injection into the skin, similar to the TB vaccine and TB test, as opposed to the standard injection into the recipient's muscle. The intradermal route of administration attempts to take advantage of the fact that 25 percent of the body surface contains specialized cells that recognize foreign microbes, mobilize the immune system's T cell response, and enhance antibody production by B cells (Steinman, 2002). The high level of antibody response occurred in adults under 60, but those recipients over 60 had a less vigorous antibody response, indicating that the intradermal vaccine did not work as well. This dose-sparing technique could extend the supply of vaccine in times of vaccine production shortage or during another pandemic when the worldwide supply of vaccine, about 300 million doses, does not meet the demand.

FluMist: The live virus vaccine

In 2003 a new, improved nasal flu vaccine was brought to the marketplace. Unlike the shot, FluMist is prepared from live vaccines. The attractive sounding FluMist vaccine could be sprayed into the nose. No needle, no shot. In a trial study conducted in Switzerland, 12,582 people were offered a free flu vaccine. They could choose the injected or nasal spray vaccine. Of this study group 1,600 were vaccinated; 97 percent chose the inhaled nasal spray. Side effects occurred in 36 percent of vaccine recipients, and flu-like symptoms in 13 percent. The most severe adverse event following administration of the vaccine was facial paralysis, which occurred in 11 patients. As a result of these adverse events, the nasal spray vaccine was removed from the market in Switzerland (Sendi, 2004).

The most common side effects of the live vaccine as

recorded in five placebo-controlled studies include head-ache, cough, sore throat, muscle aches, runny nose, tired-ness, and weakness. Each of these occurred at a statistically greater rate in vaccine recipients compared to controls. In other words, the FluMist vaccine causes flu-like symp-toms. The FDA vaccine advisory committee refused to license the FluMist vaccine for the 2002 flu season because of concerns that the live viruses in the vaccine could cause pneumonia or asthma, or spread the disease to others. The committee voted ten to four against vaccine approval. In June 2003 the committee met again and finally approved the live vaccine for people between the ages of 5 and 49. The committee refused to license the vaccine for young children because safety studies found an increased rate of asthma within forty-two days of vaccination in children under 5. Like the injected vaccine, the live vaccine was not effective in people older than 50. FluMist was not licensed for adults or children with chronic disorders of the car-diovascular and pulmonary systems, including asthma; it was also prohibited from delivery to pregnant women, anyone with a chronic metabolic disease such as diabetes, and anyone with immunosuppression from underlying dis-ease or drug therapy.

Following the administration of the live FluMist vac-cine, recipients may shed viruses for up to three weeks. The

FluMist manufacturer was required to warn that recipients should avoid close contact with immunocompromised individuals for at least twenty-one days. Since complete strangers could have close contact, this warning has caused considerable confusion. In addition, many people have compromised immune systems, making them more susceptible to flu and cold viruses. Others are taking immune suppressive corticosteroids, either in pill form or by inhaler, for asthma treatment. These people could also be injured by recipients of the FluMist vaccine who shed the virus.

For the 2003–2004 flu season, 5 million doses of FluMist were produced. However, concerns over the spread of the live virus from vaccine recipients to their contacts and the high price of the vaccine ($70) led consumers to just say no. Only 450,000 doses were sold. All the rest were discarded. For the 2004–2005 flu season, FluMist's manufacturer, MedImmune, made only 1.1 million doses and reduced the cost to $24 per dose. Then, when the injected-vaccine shortage hit in October 2004, MedImmune promised to increase its production to 3 million doses. For the 2005–2006 flu season, they plan to produce up to 10 million doses of FluMist.

Part II

Treatment and Prevention

Alternative Medical Systems

Given the many problems attributed to flu shots, we are fortunate to have several alternative medical systems that can both bolster immunity and treat the flu without side effects. These alternative medical systems have the ability to prevent disease, cure many chronic illnesses, and treat the acute illnesses that come our way. Alternative medicine is useful in three situations:

- Prevention of disease and maintenance of a healthy balance in the body in relatively healthy people
- Curing chronic, recurring disease and weakened immune function
- Treatment of acute illnesses like the flu

Prevention of the flu starts with maintaining a healthy lifestyle. Even if your health is not perfect and your diet

NATURAL HEALTH CARE SYSTEMS

Homeopathic medicine: A philosophy and form of medical treatment that uses natural remedies prepared from a plant, mineral, or animal substance capable of stimulating a healing response in the body. The medicines are prepared by pharmacies under FDA supervision. Qualified practitioners hold a CCH, DHANP, DHT, or RSHom certification in classical homeopathy, though most licensed medical providers are able to prescribe homeopathic medicines within their scope of practice regardless of certification.

Naturopathic medicine: A form of natural medicine practiced by graduates of four-year naturopathic medical schools. Training includes holistic philosophy, nutrition, homeopathy, herbs, and Chinese medicine. Practitioners hold an ND degree, and should be licensed by your state's Naturopathic Medical Board.

and exercise program not superb, you can still take supplements that increase the strength of the immune system, especially during the winter months when viruses abound. When illness strikes, you will be served best by obtaining a reliable medical diagnosis and by seeking alternative medical care. Holistic physicians, naturopathic physicians, and other holistic primary care providers are qualified to accomplish both tasks.

NATURAL HEALTH CARE SYSTEMS

Oriental medicine: The use of herbs, acupuncture, acupressure, and Oriental massage to create energetic balance in the body, practiced in accordance with principles developed in China and Tibet. Practitioners hold a Licensed Acupuncturist (Lac) and/or Doctor of Oriental Medicine (OMD) degree, and should be licensed by your state's Acupuncture Board.

Chiropractic and osteopathic manipulation: Two systems of body work that rely on manipulation of the spine and soft tissue to create balance in the body. Many practitioners also prescribe nutritional supplements and other forms of natural treatment. Every state has its own licensing board for these doctors.

The medical systems described and recommended in this book have the ability to treat acute infections with confidence. These alternative systems also share the advantage of treating viral or bacterial illness equally well. The most effective treatment programs for the flu are homeopathic medicine and herbal medicine, and the treatment sections in Parts III and IV focus primarily on their use. Consulting an expert practitioner is the ideal, and referral directories can be found in the Resources. For the many readers who do not have access to a qualified alternative medicine practitioner and must rely on their own devices to treat the flu, this book includes instructions for treating the flu at home.

Homeopathy

Homeopathy is the science and art of prescribing a highly diluted medicine prepared by a homeopathic pharmacy and made from a plant, animal, or mineral source. The medicines have no side effects or potential for toxicity. Homeopathic medical care establishes an optimum level of health in the body. It avoids the toxic and suppressive effects of drugs, and it provides curative treatment for a wide range of both chronic and acute illnesses. Homeopathic treatment has the ability to relieve symptoms at the same time that it reestablishes a healthy balance of body functions. The result of homeopathic care is a stronger constitution able to recover more quickly from future illness. Homeopathy is ultimately preventive in nature because the correctly prescribed medicine stimulates and encourages the body's innate healing abilities, creating more resistance and resilience to stress.

Many families rely on homeopathy as their primary form of health care, reserving conventional treatment for times when physical medicine is appropriate (injuries) or potentially serious medical conditions may require intervention with drugs or surgery. Nearly all acute illnesses such as flu, colds, bronchitis, and other common infections can be managed effectively with homeopathic treatment.

Homeopathic medicines are prescribed for a symptom "picture," rather than an individual symptom. Someone with a fever, chills, and diarrhea will need a different medicine than someone else with fever, heat, and headache. From a homeopathic perspective, the complex of symptoms characterizes the flu state in that person at any one time and will describe the correct homeopathic medicine. Match the symptom picture of the medicine to the symptoms of the illness and you have found the correct prescription. Finding the right homeopathic medicine for the flu is usually straightforward because the symptoms tend to be dramatic and easily characterized.

Most flu seasons and epidemics fit a common homeopathic picture, so that the majority of people with the flu will benefit from the epidemic medicine. Homeopaths in practice will easily discover this medicine in their community after seeing a few cases of the flu. For example, the epidemic medicine for the 1918 Spanish flu was *Gelsemium* (with *Bryonia* and *Eupatorium* as secondary prescriptions), which has also been the appropriate medicine for many other flu seasons. To view a database for epidemic medicines in various parts of the United States reported by experienced homeopathic practitioners, go to the flu section at www.cure-guide.com. Find your area of the country and you will see the most frequently prescribed homeopathic medicine for the flu where you live.

Homeopaths are singularly confident about treating viral illness, including flu. There is a long history of successful management of serious acute infections with homeopathy, particularly the flu. Homeopathic medicine proved extremely effective in the management of the 1918 flu epidemic, and it will prove itself in any future flu pandemic, just as it does every winter in the treatment of that year's flu cases. The Spanish flu pandemic was a plague that exceeded the ravages of the Bubonic Plague of 1347, which killed a third of the European population. Worldwide the Spanish flu killed an estimated 40 million people. In some primitive cultures the death rate was 100 percent. Fortunately, many patients in the United States had access to homeopathic medical care. A report to the American Institute of Homeopathy in 1921 documented the dramatic success of homeopathy in the worst flu pandemic in history. The death rate of 24,000 flu cases under conventional medical care in that study was 28.2 percent, while the death rate of 26,000 cases treated with homeopathy was a nearly miraculous 1.05 percent. Similarly, many homeopathic physicians each reported treating thousands of patients with very few deaths (Perko, 1999).

One specific homeopathic medicine used to treat the flu has been subjected to clinical trials. The medicine is a homeopathic preparation of the liver and heart of a Barbary duck (trade name *Oscillococcinum*, a proprietary preparation by Boiron laboratories). This medicine was first formulated in 1925. Its name arose from a spurious notion that the blood of flu victims in the 1918 pandemic contained bacteria composed of balls (cocci) that vibrated, or oscillated. Joseph Roy, a French physician of the time, identified this supposed pathogen and found it in many animal species. He chose as the source of his homeopathic preparation a duck, possibly an extremely fortuitous accident because of the association between human flu epidemics and bird viruses.

Oscillococcinum was first studied in France during the 1987 flu epidemic caused by an H1N1 virus. This multicenter study examined the effect of *Oscillococcinum* (200C) on the early symptoms of flu. Results were published in the peer-reviewed *British Journal of Clinical Pharmacology.* A group of 149 non-homeopathic physicians enlisted 487 patients in the study; each patient had developed flu-like symptoms during the previous twenty-four hours. Symptoms met strict criteria for the level of fever and the presence of associated flu symptoms. This took place in the midst of a documented flu epidemic. A treatment group and control group were established and the medicine prescribed in five doses, once at the physician's office and then twice a day for two days following. More patients in the treatment group recovered completely in the first forty-eight hours than in the control group (17 percent of patients with active treatment, compared to 10 percent of controls). This was deemed a statistically significant difference. More patients in the treatment group also judged the treatment as favorable compared to the placebo, 61 percent versus 49 percent (Ferley, 1989).

In 1990 German physicians replicated the French study of *Oscillococcinum*. They used the same criteria as the previous study and enrolled 372 patients. After forty-eight hours of treatment with *Oscillococcinum* the treatment group had significantly milder symptoms than the control group, and the number of patients with no symptoms from day two onward was significantly greater in the treatment group (17.4 percent), compared to the control group (6.6 percent) (Papp, 1998).

Both of these studies show a significant curative effect of a homeopathic medicine in the treatment of flu in carefully conducted, double-blind, placebo-controlled clinical trials. The two studies were done in different countries, each with many participating physicians, and during two different flu epidemics, presumably caused by different viruses. Conventional antiviral drugs reduce the duration of flu by about one day if taken within the first forty-eight hours of illness (Cooper, 2003). Comparing the results of these studies with the meager effect of conventional treatment shows that homeopathy carries the potential to make a dramatic difference in any flu epidemic without the risk of drug side effects.

Traditionally, homeopathic practitioners treat flu symptoms with an individual medicine that is indicated, based on the specific presenting symptoms of the patient. Homeopathic practitioners are well versed in the treatment of the flu, and the homeopathic literature of flu treatment is classic and voluminous. Most practitioners would assume that the more accurate and targeted homeopathic medicine that corresponds closely to a patient's symptoms during the flu will have a much higher cure rate than a routinely prescribed medicine utilized in studies like those of *Oscillococcinum*. Homeopaths have managed, recorded, and verified their treatment of the flu over the past 200 years (Perko, 1999).

Homeopathy is practiced by professional homeopaths, medical doctors, naturopathic physicians, acupuncturists, osteopaths, chiropractors, and nurses. Most of these professions have their own homeopathic professional associations. The Council for Homeopathic Certification (CHC) is a national board that tests and certifies practitioners in homeopathy, awarding the Certificate of Classical Homeopathy (CCH) after a rigorous examination process. The CHC publishes a directory of certified homeopaths at www.homeopathicdirectory.com, and that board coordinates certification efforts with other professional organizations, the American Board of Homeotherapeutics (ABHt), the Homeopathic Academy of Naturopathic Physicians (HANP), and the North American Society of Homeopaths (NASH). The National Center for Homeopathy also coordinates a referral directory at www.homeopathic.org.

HOME PRESCRIBING

Not everyone will have access to a homeopathic practitioner. There is also a long history of home prescribing in homeopathy, and many guides have been published instructing the lay public in how to use homeopathic medicines at home for a variety of acute illnesses, including the flu. The medicines are completely safe and nontoxic, making homeopathy a perfect choice for first-aid for your family. Home prescribing books cover a wide range of conditions in children and adults. Some of the best of these are listed in the Resources.

Parts III and IV of this book provide specific instructions for prescribing homeopathic medicines for the flu at home. These represent the first line of defense against flu outbreaks. If symptoms are not resolving in a timely manner, then consult with a knowledgeable homeopathic practitioner.

Here are some general suggestions for you to use homeopathic medicines at home to treat the flu. The choice of the medicine is of primary importance. The medicine's strength or potency, the dosage, and the frequency of repetition are of negligible importance. Any strength is likely to work. The strength is measured by the number of times the medicine has been subjected to the homeopathic pharmaceutical process. Strength of homeopathic medicines is expressed in terms of X (as in 6X) or C (as in 12C). The C, or centesimal, range of potencies is stronger than the X, or decimal, range, and a higher number indicates a stronger or more deep-acting form of the medicine. Using homeopathic medicines in a 30C strength is usually sufficient for acute flu illnesses, and these are available at larger health food stores. A 6X or 12C medicine is likely to work just as well, and strengths ranging as high as 200 or 1,000 (1M) are frequently used by homeopathic practitioners. Similarly, the dosage is unimportant. A homeopathic medicine will work if you give one pellet or five. There is absolutely no toxicity involved, and a child can safely eat the contents of an entire bottle of homeopathic medicine with no untoward effects. One dose of a medicine is just as likely to work as taking it three times per day or every two hours. In general, once a homeopathic medicine is acting beneficially, it is wise to stop and not continue repetitions. On the other hand, children tend to burn off the effect of a homeopathic medicine during an illness, so it makes sense to repeat the dose several times a day until symptoms are clearly improved. For an illness with more force and more dramatic symptoms, a higher strength is indicated and more repetitions are appropriate, even in adults. For most slow-paced flu illnesses, three doses per day is usually adequate given the *proviso* that once symptoms clearly improve, it is wise to stop and wait. Repeating the medicine later if symptoms return is always an option. For severe symptoms, homeopaths may repeat even a high strength of a medicine every half hour.

If a medicine is not working, then consider either consulting a more detailed homeopathic home prescribing book to find a medicine more closely aligned with the presenting symptoms, or consult with a homeopathic professional. Complications of the flu need to be treated by an experienced homeopathic practitioner. Anyone with a deep, productive cough with fever or shortness of breath should consult a medical provider.

Over-the-counter combination homeopathic remedies defy the basic homeopathic tenet of treating the individual with the most accurate prescription. These medicines are found in health food stores and pharmacies labeled *flu* or *colds* or *cough*. The theory behind these combinations is the shotgun approach: Throw several typically indicated medicines at a symptom and see if something works. If the correct medicine is not present, then no beneficial effect will occur. Experienced homeopaths also notice a disorganizing effect from taking many different homeopathic medicines in combination.

Acupuncture and Oriental medicine

Oriental medicine encompasses several medical systems with a common origin and similar philosophy—traditional Chinese medicine, Tibetan medicine, Japanese acupuncture, and Korean acupuncture. Since traditional Chinese medicine (TCM) is by far the most common form in the U.S., Oriental medicine in this book is assumed to be TCM. Acupuncturists are licensed in most states and they are trained and board certified in the use of acupuncture as well as Chinese herbal medicine. Other medical providers (naturopathic physicians and medical doctors) may also specialize in Oriental medicine after appropriate training.

Oriental medicine has evolved into a complete system of healing through continuous practice and experimentation over 2,500 years. Chinese medical philosophy views the human body as a dynamic organism animated by a vital energy known as *Qi* (pronounced chee), which is in a constantly shifting balance. When this energy is harmoniously regulated, health and vigor are preserved. When the vital energy is disturbed, the organ systems of the body cease to function smoothly and symptoms arise. Disturbances can arise from external environmental influences, internal imbalances, or the effects of unhealthy habits of living.

Oriental medicine has a long and distinguished history of treating infectious diseases. The theory of Oriental medicine describes the stages of acute illnesses in exhaustive detail, and each stage and type of illness has a specific treatment protocol using Chinese herbs and/or acupuncture therapy. Licensed acupuncturists are trained and qualified to manage a variety of infectious illnesses, including the various stages and complications of the flu.

Chinese medicine views the flu as an attack by pathogenic Wind and Heat. The Heat symptoms include those of the inflammatory response—fever, sore throat, and dry cough. Wind symptoms manifest as joint pain, headache, and aching muscles. Typically, a treatment for flu in Oriental medicine consists of an herbal formula prepared from individual herbs that clear Heat and dispel Wind from the body. One of the most famous of these formulas is *Yin Chiao San,* a remedy that was developed at the end of the eighteenth century. Modern formulations of *Yin Chiao* (also *Yin Qiao*) are produced by numerous mainland Chinese and American companies and are increasingly available in large health and natural food stores. These formulations are produced in pill form as well as concentrated, liquid extracts. The name *Yin Chiao* derives from the formula's two main ingredients, *Jin **Yin** Hua* (Lonicera, honeysuckle flowers) and *Lian **Qiao*** (forsythia buds), both of which clear Wind and Heat. Various manufacturers modify the original formula for specific effects, but the basic ingredients serve the function of clearing Heat and expelling Wind, thus relieving the cough, sore throat, headache, body ache, and fever that signal the onset of a flu.

Yin Chiao is most effectively used in the first stages of flu, during the first day or two when Heat symptoms predominate. This is the time when it can dramatically curtail an attack of flu. For later stages, when congestion and deeper cough are more pronounced, other formulas are more appropriate. *Yin Chiao* dispels pathogenic Wind, clears Heat, resolves toxin, benefits the throat, relieves thirst, and diffuses lung *Qi* (Fratkin, 2001).

YIN CHIAO FORMULA INGREDIENTS

Lonicera — clears Wind and Heat
Forsythia — clears Wind and Heat
Lophatherum — clears Heat
Schizonepeta — expels Wind
Arctium — disperses Wind and Heat and benefits the throat
Platycodon — relieves cough by opening the lungs and expelling phlegm
Mentha — clears the head (headache) and benefits the throat
Glycine Soja — releases the exterior
Glycyrrhiza — harmonizes other herbs and stops coughing

Gan Mao Ling, a remedy that was developed in the last fifty years, is another well-known formula for flu characterized by sinus congestion, yellow nasal discharge, chills, stiff neck and back, sore throat, and swollen glands. The primary ingredients are *Ilex pubescens* and *Evodia rutecarpa,* both of which have strong antiviral effects.

Zhong Gan Ling is a formula for full-blown influenza, after the initial Wind and Heat attack. Now the symptoms are proceeding into serious muscle aching, especially in the neck and shoulders, and increased fever. It is a strong formula for relieving high fever and treating cough with thick phlegm. The *Zhong Gan Ling* formula dispels path-

GAN MAO LING FORMULA INGREDIENTS

Ilex—antiviral
Evodia—antiviral
Chrysanthemum—disperses Wind and clears Heat
Vitex—disperses Wind and clears Heat
Isatis—drains Heat
Lonicera—clears Wind and Heat

ZHONG GAN LING FORMULA INGREDIENTS

Ilex—antiviral, cleanses pathogens, opens blood circulation
Pueraria—releases the muscles and clears Heat
Verbena—clears Heat and drains dampness (congestion, phlegm)
Isatis—drains Heat
Artemesia—clears Heat
Gypsum—drains fire, clears Heat from the lungs
Notopterygium—disperses cold, releases the exterior, relieves head-ache and muscle aches

ogenic Wind, clears Heat, resolves toxins, cools the blood, and moistens the throat (Fratkin, 2001).

Several U.S. herbal manufacturers have adapted these formulas that treat the flu and are producing their own versions of the classic formulations, sometimes adding other ingredients. Health Concerns (Isatis Gold), Chinese Modular Solutions (Purge External Wind, Purge Heat, Bug Beater, Chill Chaser), Seven Forests (Ilex 15), Kan Traditionals (*Zhong Gan Ling*), Jade Dragon (*Yin Qiao, Gan Mao Ling*), and many others produce similar formulas.

Acupuncture treatment offers many important strategies for building the body's defenses, thwarting the pathogenic factors that contribute to flu symptoms and relieving specific symptoms. Specific combinations of acupuncture points are selected for relieving headache and sore throats, reducing fever, relieving respiratory congestion, and subduing cough. Acupuncture is usually employed in combination with herbs to restore harmony and promote a vigorous defense against invasions from pathogens and the external factors of wind, heat, and cold. The goal of acupuncture is always to promote or invigorate the circulation of vital energy and to harmonize the interaction of the organ systems.

Acupuncture and Chinese herbal medicine provide many tools for optimizing immune function and improving overall resistance to stress and illness. An acupuncturist will usually prescribe an herbal formula intended to confer immune-system-enhancing effects for anyone with weakened resistance and recurrent infections. Various formulas are designed for children and adults and for different types of chronic problems. In addition, correcting any specific imbalance with either acupuncture or herbal medicine will strengthen the body, helping to maintain optimum balance and immunity. The result is invigorated body functions and a more vibrant state of health.

Western herbs

Two herbs have proven especially effective in managing flu symptoms: echinacea and black elderberry.

Echinacea stimulates white blood cell activity (Melchart, 1995) and increases the body's production of interferon, an antiviral agent (Burger, 1997). Several studies have shown echinacea's ability to treat the flu. In a German clinical trial, a 900-mg daily dose of echinacea resulted in a significant reduction in flu symptoms, including weakness, chills, sweating, sore throat, headaches, and muscle and joint aches (Bodinet, 1993). A second study showed that echinacea tea (five to six cups per day) relieved flu symptoms in a shorter period of time, compared to a placebo (Lindenmuth, 2000).

An alternative and safe herbal treatment for the flu is **black elderberry** extract. Elderberry proved to cut short the flu by four days in a double-blind controlled study.

Nearly 90 percent of patients given elderberry extract were completely cured in two to three days, while in the control group it took six days for 90 percent of patients to recover (Zakay-Rones, 2004). A second clinical study showed similar results. Among the group receiving elderberry, 75 percent were much improved within two days, and 90 percent were completely cured by day three. The control group took six days before 90 percent were cured (Zakay-Rones, 1995). In that study elderberry was also found to inhibit the replication of both type A and type B flu viruses.

Those researchers also investigated the mode of action of elderberry on viruses. They found that elderberry inhibited the enzyme that attaches the virus to human cells and also inhibited the enzyme that breaks down the human cell wall, allowing the virus to enter and kill the cell. Another group of researchers also showed that elderberry activates the immune system by increasing inflammatory and anti-inflammatory cytokine production (Barak, 2002).

The usual preparation of elderberry is Sambucol syrup (prepared either with glucose syrup and honey, or with sorbitol). Adults take two teaspoons of syrup per day, beginning immediately at the onset of symptoms; children take one teaspoon.

Naturopathic medicine

Naturopathy is not a specific form of treatment; it is a comprehensive system of medicine with extensive training in natural therapies. Founded upon a holistic philosophy, naturopathic medicine combines safe and effective traditional therapies with the most current advances in modern medicine. Naturopathic physicians (NDs) are trained in basic medical sciences and conventional diagnostics, and their training in therapeutics includes nutrition, botanical medicine, homeopathy, natural childbirth, traditional Chinese medicine, hydrotherapy, naturopathic manipulative therapy, pharmacology, and minor surgery. Often a naturopathic physician will specialize in one or more of these treatment modalities. The goal of a naturopathic physician is to employ therapies that support and promote the body's natural healing process, using a holistic approach to health that integrates the healing powers of body, mind, and spirit. Naturopathic physicians are well-trained in the various modalities that successfully treat the flu—homeopathy, Chinese herbs, and Western herbs.

Currently, thirteen states and the District of Columbia have licensing laws for naturopathic doctors. In these states, naturopathic doctors are required to graduate from a four-year, residential naturopathic medical school and pass an extensive post-doctoral board examination (NPLEX) to receive their license. Naturopathic physicians are primary care and specialty doctors with a broad scope of practice. They are highly trained in both assessing and treating disease, but they also address the underlying cause of disease through effective, individualized natural therapies.

Prevention
Homeopathy

For at least the past 150 years, homeopathic practitioners have used the medicine *Influenzinum* as a flu preventive. *Influenzinum* is a homeopathic medicine made from flu viruses. A proprietary preparation is produced by Dolisos pharmacy each year, using the flu virus strains recommended by the World Health Organization for the year's vaccine production (*Dolivaxil*—containing *Influenzinum* 9C). The typical dosage is once per week for four weeks beginning in October or later, followed by another dose three weeks later.

Between the years 1918 and 1957, the preparation of *Influenzinum* was derived from samples of blood or nasal secretions taken from patients who contracted the flu during the deadly 1918 flu pandemic. Since 1957 *Influenzinum* preparations have come from a homeopathic preparation of the yearly flu viruses chosen for the flu vaccine.

In 1998 the French Society of Homeopathy conducted a survey of twenty-three homeopathic doctors concerning their use of *Influenzinum* as a flu preventive (Coulamy, 1998). The survey included use of *Influenzinum* over a ten-year period (1987–1998) in 453 patients. The protocol for the frequency of doses varied considerably among these doctors. Weekly doses were used by 26 percent of participants and monthly dosage by 23 percent. Another 16 percent used a weekly then monthly dosage plan, and 35 percent applied some other dosage protocol. For 80 percent of respondents, treatment began in the fall (September through November) and ended between February and April. In this French survey, 70 percent of participants used a 9C strength of *Influenzinum*. (In the U.S. practitioners often use a higher strength because of the different prescribing preferences between the two countries.)

Results of the survey were remarkable. In approximately 90 percent of the cases, no instances of the flu occurred when *Influenzinum* was used preventively, no matter what dosage protocol was used. The physicians deemed the effectiveness good to very good in 90 percent of the cases. In 5 percent there was no protective effect. Of the patients, 98 percent expressed a desire to take the same preventive treatment the following year. Certainly this confidence in homeopathic prevention among physicians with many years of experience and their patients speaks to the effectiveness of *Influenzinum* as a flu preventive. It should be noted that a clinical study that approaches statistical significance evaluating the preventive effects of any homeopathic preparation would probably be prohibitively expensive.

Chiropractic manipulation

(Contributed by Jeanne Ohm, DC, Executive Coordinator, International Chiropractic Pediatric Association)

Chiropractic care is not the treatment of disease. Rather, it removes spinal nerve stress, a serious and often painless condition that most children and adults have in their bodies. Spinal nerve stress interferes with the proper functioning of the nervous system. It also can weaken internal organs and organ systems, lower resistance, reduce healing potential, and set the stage for reduced immune function and respiratory system weakness—all of which can create the perfect setting for a severe bout of flu and its complications.

When a chiropractor frees the nervous system from spinal stress, the healing power of the body is unleashed—the immune system functions more efficiently, resistance to disease increases, and the body functions more efficiently. Your body can then respond to internal and external environmental stresses such as germs, changes in temperature, humidity, toxins, pollen, and emotional stresses with greater efficiency.

Spinal nerve stress (also referred to as vertebral subluxations, the subluxation complex, or "pinched nerves") is a misalignment or distortion of the spinal column, skull, hips, and related tissues (the structural system) that irritates, stretches, impinges, or otherwise interferes with the proper function of the nervous system (brain, spinal cord, spinal nerves, and outlying or peripheral nerves). Since the nervous system controls the function of the body, any interference can have wide-ranging effects.

Spinal nerve stress can be caused by physical, chemical, and/or emotional stress. Physical stress may start in the womb, with the baby lying in a distorted or twisted manner. Spinal nerve stress in newborns is more common than previously realized. This may be caused by a traumatic or difficult birth, which can introduce great stress to the infant's skull, spinal column, and pelvis. Throughout childhood, the normal childhood traumas every child experiences can be a source of spinal and cranial trauma. Most of the time, the pain from the initial injury "goes away"; however, the damage continues to affect the future function of the child's nerve system. In addition, adults suffer many injuries, occupational physical stresses, and postural problems that all have effect on spinal alignment.

Chiropractic doctors can correct spinal nerve stress. This is accomplished first by analyzing the spinal column and related structures for balance and proper function. Where the spinal column is found to be functioning improperly, the Doctor of Chiropractic (DC) performs precise corrective procedures called spinal adjustments. When chiropractors use their hands and/or specialized instruments to gently and specifically correct those abnormal areas, the spine and cranium regain their intended state of balance and the nerve system is freed from stress.

Osteopathic manipulation

Doctors of osteopathy (DO) are fully licensed physicians able to prescribe pharmaceutical drugs, perform surgery, and attend births. What distinguishes them from MDs is their extensive training in osteopathic manipulative treatment (OMT). DOs use their hands during OMT to diagnose injury and illness, giving special attention to the joints, bones, muscles, and nerves. Manipulations improve circulation, which in turn creates a normal nerve and blood supply, enabling the body to heal itself.

OMT is a highly developed and sophisticated method of body work that may include a wide range of techniques. Cranial osteopathy is a specific approach within the osteopathic concept. It influences the structure and fluid surrounding the central nervous system, creating an impact on the total body and initiating the body's inherent capacity to heal itself. Visceral manipulation relates to the interrelationship of the structure and function of the internal organs. Manipulation of the viscera can benefit a variety of internal organ dysfunctions including respiratory problems and immune system weakness. Other specific osteopathic techniques include myofascial release, lymphatic drainage, and somatoemotional release, among many others. These physical and energetic manipulations provide potent stimulation to the body's own healing mechanisms, resulting in a higher state of balance and greater equilibrium—and enabling a more efficient immune response to the flu and its potentially serious complicating infections.

Body movement therapies

A multitude of body movement practices have a positive impact on health, creating harmony and balance in the body and a strong immune system capable of overcoming respiratory infections and the flu. These practices include the many Indian systems of yoga, the Chinese systems of *tai chi* and *chi gong*, the Japanese system of *Aikido*, the Alexander technique, and the Feldenkrais technique's awareness through movement lessons.

Explore these mind-body movement practices and find the one that resonates with your own cultural orientation, intuition, and beliefs. Find the practice that feels right to you and integrate it into your daily life and exercise routines. Each of them has the potential to build a stronger immune system, increase respiratory capacity and strength of the respiratory system, and help with self-healing. See the Resources for information sources.

Dietary guidelines

The best type of diet to maintain healthy immune function and avoid the flu is actually quite simple: Eat lots of fresh fruits and vegetables. Avoid pesticides whenever possible by eating organic foods. Get vitamin A from meats, eggs, and butter. One of the most important dietary issues for healthy cell function and a robust immune system is maintaining the correct balance of fats in the body. Get omega-3 fats from fish oil supplements and animal products, eat saturated fats, and remove all trans-fats from your diet. At least 50 percent of dietary fat should be saturated (Watkins, 1996). Omega-3 fats are retained better in tissues in the presence of saturated fats, and saturated fats promote healthy immune systems because of their anti-microbial properties that prevent the build-up of harmful microorganisms in the digestive tract. Contrary to accepted beliefs, saturated fats do not cause heart disease; they prevent heart disease and cancer.

Trans-fats damage cell membranes, block the utilization of essential fatty acids, and promote disease (diabetes, heart disease, immune system dysfunction, and allergies). They are artificially manufactured as partially hydrogenated oils. You will find them in most packaged foods down the center aisles of the supermarket, in chips, crackers, breads, cakes, croissants, and cookies. Trans-fats sit in cell membranes, creating a barrier that blocks the exchange of nutrients that promote health and chemicals necessary for efficient cell function. Trans-fats promote inflammation in cells and create an environment that makes mucous membranes more susceptible to irritation, allergic reactions, and infection.

Avoid meats with nitrates, nitrites, growth hormones, and antibiotics. Eat range-fed beef and organic, cage-free chickens and their eggs. Use organic dairy products. Never eat aspartame (Nutrasweet, Equal) or saccharine (Sweet'n Low).

Avoid high-fructose corn syrup, which is used as a sweetener in many packaged foods. Corn syrup is convenient for food manufacturers because it retains moisture and blends well with other ingredients, but the free fructose in corn syrup interferes with the heart's use of minerals and depletes the ability of white blood cells to defend against infections.

Avoid soy products. Soy interferes with calcium, magnesium, zinc, and iron absorption, all of which are necessary for healthy immune system function to defend the body against infections like the flu. Phytic acid blocks the uptake of essential minerals in the intestinal tract, and soy has one of the highest phytic acid levels of any grain or legume (Reddy, 2002). Only fermentation of soy products in the preparation of miso, soy sauce, and tempeh removes the phytates responsible for mineral depletion.

Here are some further suggestions for adults. Take a supplement of omega-3 fats in the form of fish oil, cod liver oil (totaling 1,000–2,000 mg EPA, eicosapentaenoic acid), or an algae DHA source capsule (Neuromins, 200 mg DHA, docosahexaenoic acid). Take vitamin E as d-alpha tocopherol or a mixed tocopherol (400 IU). Eat fruits and vegetables high in antioxidants—tomatoes, broccoli, red or black beans, blueberries, apples, grapes, and seeds. Eat fruits that contain vitamin C—oranges, grapefruit, kiwi, berries, mango, papaya, pineapple, and watermelon.

Adults should also avoid a diet high in starches in the form of wheat products, bread, pasta, and potatoes. Don't eat foods sweetened with sugar. All of these products stimulate insulin production, insulin reactions, low blood sugar, and heart disease. For specific suggestions about supplements that build immune function in children and adults, see Parts III and IV of this book.

Part III

Children
Prevention
Breastfeeding

Breast milk provides the best immune system protection possible for your child. The immune-enhancing power of breast milk is truly amazing. Many studies have shown that breast milk prevents infection, decreases the severity of illnesses, and promotes a strong immune system response that also prevents complications of acute diseases. Breastfeeding infants have fewer ear infections, diarrheal illnesses, respiratory infections, and allergies, and a lower rate of asthma (Oddy, 2004). Continue breastfeeding for at least six to twelve months if possible to ensure the maximum protection for complications from flu symptoms. Studies have also shown that the longer you breastfeed, the more protective the effect of breast milk, and this protection will persist even long after children are weaned (Hanson, 1998).

Many specific substances contained in breast milk provide immune enhancement and actual immunity to disease. Immunoglobulins in human milk provide passive protection from pathogenic microorganisms. White blood cells in human milk will actively ingest bacteria and viruses that invade your infant's body. In addition, lymphocytes (a type of white blood cell) carrying specific antibodies pass through breast milk to your baby. Several other chemicals in breast milk (lactoferrin and lysozyme) protect the breastfeeding child from infection by destroying or inhibiting growth of bacteria (Goldman, 1982). Many other resistance factors in breast milk (including interferon) help the child's developing immune system function (Chandra, 1978). These protective effects are especially important in flu illnesses because of the risk of complications caused by bacteria.

Colostrum

The immune-enhancing effects of breast milk can be continued in older children by giving them cow's colostrum as a nutritional supplement. The first food a newborn baby receives is colostrum, the clear or yellowish thick fluid secreted from a mother's breasts after childbirth. Colostrum transmits to babies antibodies and other immune-enhancing substances that actively prevent infections and stimulate the immune system.

Colostrum contains immune defense factors. The most prominent of these factors is an immunoglobulin, IgA, which resides on mucous membranes such as the intestinal lining and protects the body from invading microorganisms. Colostrum, like breast milk, contains white blood cells that ingest bacteria and release IgA. Lactoferrin prevents bacteria from reproducing. Lysozyme destroys microorganisms on contact. Cytokines regulate the intensity and duration of immune responses, boosting T-cell activity and stimulating production of protective immunoglobulins. Specific sugars, including oligo polysaccharides and glycoconjugates, bind to bacteria that typically cause ear infections, lung infections, and diarrhea, and block their attachment to mucous membranes. All of these powerful immune defense factors are available in one simple supplement.

Children can take bovine colostrum as a supplement throughout the entire flu season. You can obtain colostrum in powder, chewable flavored tablets, or capsules. Children under the age of 6 can take at least one-half teaspoon of colostrum powder or two tablets or capsules. Children over 6 should take one teaspoon of powder or three to four tablets or capsules.

Nutrition in older children

Good nutrition lays the groundwork for a strong immune system in your child. This includes reliance upon natural foods, and avoidance of chemicals and refined products. Fresh fruits and vegetables provide essential nutrients for the growing child, including antioxidants and vitamin C. Processed foods such as canned vegetables and jars of baby food have fewer vitamins and altered forms of essential nutrients.

Vitamin A is needed for proper mucous membrane function. It is essential for the growth and repair of body tissues, and for efficient digestion of protein. Vitamin A promotes good eyesight, strong bones and teeth, and a vital immune system. White blood cells, T-lymphocytes, and every cell in the important mucosal barriers of the respiratory, digestive, and urinary tracts require vitamin A.

A diet containing significant amounts of fat will help ensure adequate vitamin A intake. Whole-milk products, butter, and free-range eggs will help maintain necessary levels of this important nutrient. Use organic sources. For those who may not be getting enough vitamin A, a supplement is essential.

The recommended daily amount (RDA) of vitamin A is 3,000 IU per day for adults (reduced from 5,000 IU) and

1,000–2,000 IU for children, depending on their age (1,000 at age 1, 2,000 by age 9). Primitive diets probably maintained ten times that amount. One egg contains 300 IU of vitamin A; one cup of whole milk or whole-milk yogurt contains 225–250 IU, and one tablespoon of butter contains 350 IU. The amount of vitamin A may vary by the season and the feed of the animals.

Most children would benefit from a vitamin A supplement derived from fish oil. One tablespoon of cod liver oil contains at least 3,000 IU of A. Proper dosage is one teaspoon per fifty pounds of body weight. Several studies have also shown that vitamin A supplements during viral illnesses promote rapid recovery and prevent complications. Children can take 1,000 to 5,000 IU of vitamin A derived from fish oil without any problem.

Nutritional supplements

Children can take a few simple, specific supplements to maintain a strong and vital immune system during the fall and winter months when colds and flus predominate.

An omega-3 fat supplement in the form of fish oil capsules, DHA from algae (Neuromins), or cod liver oil will establish healthy cell membranes that prevent inflammation and resist toxins and attack by pathogens. One teaspoon of cod liver oil or 200 mg of DHA for each fifty pounds of body weight is an appropriate dose.

Vitamin E will ensure that fatty acids are maintained at optimum efficiency once they are absorbed into cells. In addition, vitamin E has anti-inflammatory effects and increases resistance to infection. Use only natural vitamin E (d-alpha-tocopherol), not the synthetic form (dl-alpha-tocopherol). A mixed tocopherol form of vitamin E is best because children need the gamma as well as the alpha forms. An appropriate dose is 100 IU for children under 2 and 200 IU for children age 2–12.

Zinc stimulates immune function, prevents infections, and acts as a cofactor in many enzyme reactions, including the creation of antioxidants. Normal dosage is 10–20 mg per day. If zinc supplementation is continued over a prolonged period of time, it should be given in conjunction with copper in a ratio of ten to one to prevent copper deficiency.

Vitamin C has anti-inflammatory effects, antioxidant activity, and antibiotic qualities. A daily supplement of vitamin C during the winter months will round out the immune system prevention program. Use 500 mg for children under 3 years old and 1,000 mg for older children.

The easiest way to give supplements to children is through powdered sources mixed in a blender with fruit,

IMMUNE SUPPLEMENTS FOR CHILDREN—DAILY DOSAGE		
	1- to 2-year-olds	3- to 12-year-olds
Cod liver oil	1 teaspoon per 50 pounds weight (both age groups)	
Or DHA from algae (Neuromins) or fish oil	100 mg	250 mg
Colostrum	½ teaspoon powder	1 teaspoon powder
Zinc	10 mg	20 mg
Copper	1 mg	2 mg
Vitamin E (d-alpha-tocopherol or mixed tocopherols)	100 IU	200 IU
Vitamin C	500 mg	1,000 mg

fruit juice, yogurt or milk (rice milk for younger children and children with milk sensitivities), and honey (for children over 12 months old). Capsules can be opened and dumped into the blender. Children can chew oil-based supplements in soft gels or you can stick a pin into them and squirt out the contents onto something they will eat.

Treatment

SICK AND TIRED

Amy was sick and tired. Her daughter Samantha was perfectly happy and healthy until she turned 1 in October. It was February and there was no end in sight for the constant barrage of infections, fevers, and cough that had plagued her daughter all winter. It all began innocently enough with a runny nose, fever, and fussiness at night. Alarmed that it could be an ear infection, Amy dutifully took Samantha to the doctor. She was right. Mother's intuition, such a wonderful thing. We'll just give her a course of antibiotics, said the amiable pediatrician. Should get her good as new in a few days. It did. Then one week later, Samantha had the runny nose again. This time it ran green in a few days and every night Amy and Samantha were both awakened many times by the baby's choking cough. Amy Googled "nighttime cough" and called the doctor again, this time worried about bronchitis and allergies. Just a sinus infection, said the doctor. Antibiotics will take care of that. More pink medicine.

The green goop went away, but the cough never disappeared. By early December Samantha was taking longer naps, looking tired, eating less, and often cranky. What happened to Amy's shining, happy girl? Then Samantha developed low-grade fevers off and on. The pediatrician patiently explained that this was Samantha's first winter without the benefit of her mother's protective antibodies. She needed to build her own antibodies by fighting off the germs in her environment. It was common for children this age to get eight colds per year. It did not help that Samantha's older sister brought home cold viruses from school. Yes, but what about the infections and the antibiotics? What do they have to do with colds? The pediatrician assured Amy that Samantha was fine. He had his hand on the doorknob, the definitive signal of the busy doctor with no time for small talk.

Amy stopped going to the pediatrician about Samantha's symptoms after that. What was the point? She did her own research and began giving Samantha vitamin C. She stopped all dairy products. She was determined. Nothing helped.

Then in January Samantha came down with a high fever and a brutal, aching flu with symptoms that lasted for a week. Samantha was looking pale and withdrawn. She had dark circles under her eyes.

At the baby gymnastics class that Samantha usually missed because of illness, Amy's friend Gretchen was concerned. "She doesn't look very healthy," Gretchen observed.

"I don't know what to do," Amy responded. "She's been sick all winter."

"What about homeopathy?" Gretchen suggested.

Usually Amy tended to ignore well-meaning advice from her earth-mother type acquaintances. But Gretchen grew up in Germany where alternative medical approaches were more accepted, and maybe she did have something to offer, Amy thought. Nothing that Amy was doing had helped. So Amy listened.

At the visit to the homeopath, Amy's anxieties about a hippy enclave were quickly relieved. The office was comfortable and inviting, with a professional but friendly atmosphere that immediately put her child at ease. Samantha plopped onto the floor and began playing with the toys, hardly her typical reaction at the pediatrician's office.

The homeopath explained that her approach was holistic. She discovered that Samantha sweated on her head during sleep, and her feet got sweaty during the day, that she was shy and slow to warm up in new situations, a little clingy, but very bright. She craved ice and salt. All of this seemed mysteriously important to the homeopath.

Finally, she gave her pronouncement. Samantha's system was disordered by the antibiotics. She needed a probiotic supplement to replace the intestinal bacteria destroyed by antibiotics and a homeopathic constitutional medicine,

Silica. *Colostrum would help too. This program would reestablish a normal balance in her system and make sure that Samantha's immune system became vigorous and resilient.*

Amy listened doubtfully, but decided the program was harmless, and what other choice did she have? Just as Gretchen predicted when she suggested Amy try a different approach, Samantha's energy improved, her normal color returned, and the gray circles disappeared. The runny nose never came back, and no signs of the cough. Samantha cruised through the rest of the winter and spring in perfect health.

Some special issues apply to children with the flu. First, children can develop high fevers with much less severe accompanying symptoms than adults. A child with a 104°F (40°C) temperature is miserable, but can also quickly rally. An adult with this level of fever feels as if he will die. Second, because children have easily weakened digestive functions, they tend to develop more digestive symptoms than adults. They often have vomiting and diarrhea with the flu, sometimes as one of the first few symptoms of illness. Third, children go through stages of the flu fairly quickly and the treatment regimen may need to change frequently during the course of the illness to match the symptom picture. This applies especially to homeopathic medicines. A medicine that fits the picture on day one may transition to a new medicine on day two and again on day four.

Homeopathic medicines are equally and completely safe for newborns, infants, and older children. Dosage is typically one or two pellets of sugar pills that have been prepared by a homeopathic pharmacy. Infants can hold the pellets in their cheeks and they will dissolve. Older children can chew them. Alternatively, parents can crush the pellets and dissolve them in water, then give a half or whole teaspoon as a dose.

Children younger than 2 years old are more likely to develop serious complications of the flu than older children or adults if they are treated with conventional medical approaches. In one study children under 2 were twelve times as likely to be hospitalized with respiratory disease during the flu season, compared to children over 5 years of age (Izurieta, 2000). In a second study children under 1 suffered significantly more complications of heart and lung problems, compared to older children and adults (Neuzil, 2000). These alarming statistics from conventional medicine should encourage all parents to seek alternative care for their children who encounter the flu.

A note about fever

Fevers, or elevated temperatures, are good. Fever is the body's mechanism of fighting infections, speeding up metabolism to increase heart rate and increasing the blood supply where it is needed, producing more white blood cells to devour pathogens, and increasing antibody responses to infection. Fevers should not be suppressed with fever-reducing medication (antipyretics). Acetaminophen, ibuprofen, and aspirin have no place in the home treatment of fevers below 105°F (40.5°C). Never use aspirin in viral illnesses because it could cause serious disease complications. A child with a fever above 105°F should be under medical supervision because a serious infection such as meningitis may be the cause, but only fevers above 108°F (42.2°C) have been known to cause brain damage. If your baby under 3 months of age has a fever or seems sick and lethargic, see your medical provider.

Studies have shown that depriving the body of its ability to develop a fever with antipyretics may prolong the illness, decrease antibody response, and increase the likelihood of disease complications such as pneumonia and meningitis. Medical authorities generally agree that reducing fevers interferes with immune mechanisms and worsens illness. Treating animals with antipyretics during fevers

DANGER SIGNS WITH FEVER—
SEE A MEDICAL PROVIDER

Any fever in a child under 3 months of age

Fever of 105°F (40.5°C)

Appearance and behavior: lethargic, pale skin, unresponsive, weak crying

Symptoms: repeated vomiting, severe headache, stiff neck

increases their fatality rates.

Seizures can occur with fevers. Some children are more prone to these febrile seizures, and their parents dread the onset of illness. About 50 percent of children who experience one febrile seizure will have another one in the future. Typically, a child will either begin twitching prior to the onset of a seizure, or the seizure will begin suddenly and unexpectedly. If your child begins quivering or trembling, take her into the shower with you immediately. Cooling her down may avert the onset of convulsions. Febrile seizures are frightening to parents even though they only last ten to fifteen seconds, but they do not result in any type of damage to the child. They do not proceed to later epilepsy. If a seizure occurs, keep your child upright if possible and make sure she is breathing well. Reassure her. If she vomits, turn her on her side. Call your medical provider immediately, once the seizure is over. Unless your child is choking or having difficulty breathing, it is usually not necessary to summon emergency services.

Supportive measures

Encourage your child to drink fluids. If she is vomiting, then be careful about giving more than a sip at a time. Ice chips or frozen juice popsicles work well.

Wiping children with a cool, wet washcloth will cause the water to evaporate from the skin and have a cooling effect. It may not bring down the temperature, but it does provide some relief of symptoms.

If a baby has difficulty nursing because of nasal obstruction, or an older child has trouble sleeping, take him into the bathroom and steam it up with the hot shower. Let him breathe the steam for five minutes. This will loosen phlegm and moisten the dry, irritated mucous membranes of the nose and throat. Humidifiers and vaporizers are inefficient, messy, and tend to produce and distribute mold.

Keep your child home from school and resting until twenty-four hours after a fever has subsided. Often children will have a fever in the evening, burn it off in the night, and feel much better in the morning. Then the fever may return later in the afternoon and the child feels droopy again. Better to rest until recovery is complete than to rush back to normal activities and prolong the illness.

If your child has persistent diarrhea or vomiting with the flu, you need to watch for signs of dehydration, which occurs when a child is not taking in enough fluids to compensate for the fluid loss. The essential sign of dehydration is weight loss. If your baby or child is not losing weight, dehydration is unlikely. A 5 percent loss in weight signifies moderate dehydration. A 10 percent loss in weight suggests serious dehydration and the need to seek medical attention immediately. Dehydration can lead to inability to maintain adequate blood pressure, resulting in shock. Babies with diarrhea need to be carefully monitored for signs of dehydration.

Home treatment for diarrhea consists of giving a probiotic intestinal bacteria supplement containing *Lactobacillus acidophilus* and *L. bifidus*, a homeopathic medicine, plus an electrolyte solution if signs of dehydration occur (either Pedialyte or a homemade rehydrating electrolyte solution). Children often refuse Pedialyte because of the taste. If you make your own rehydrating solution, you can add a small portion of fruit juice or fruit syrup to the formula. These solutions should only be used if dehydration occurs.

SIGNS OF DEHYDRATION

Weight loss

Dry mouth and absence of tears

Skin feels dry and doughy

Eyes appear sunken

Diminished urine output

Lethargy

HOMEMADE REHYDRATION ELECTROLYTE SOLUTION

1 quart filtered or spring water

½ teaspoon table salt

½ teaspoon baking soda

8 teaspoons sugar

A probiotic supplement will help restore normal intestinal bacteria that get washed out during episodes of diarrhea. Probiotics can be purchased at any health food store. For breastfeeding babies, one-quarter teaspoon of a powdered *L. bifidus* formula is appropriate, mixed with breast milk; for older babies, mix in yogurt or applesauce. Older children should take one-quarter teaspoon of a powdered, *L. acidophilus* or combination bacteria formula. Refrigerate all probiotic supplements.

Homeopathic treatment

If a family member or a friend has exposed your child to the flu, give her *Influenzinum* (9C to 30C) as a preventive, once a week for four weeks.

If your child begins to exhibit symptoms, use the guidelines in the next sections to restore health.

FIRST STAGE OF FLU

One of three medicines will usually be indicated for the first stage of flu symptoms in children: *Belladonna, Gelsemium,* or *Arsenicum.*

Belladonna is characterized by fever without other significant symptoms except lots of heat and a headache. Usually by the time other symptoms arise, a different homeopathic medicine is indicated. Children who need *Belladonna* are usually **quite tired** and seem **dull, glassy eyed,** and **lethargic.** They tend to have a red, **flushed face,** and sometimes will also have **cool hands and feet.**

Children needing *Gelsemium* are **achy, chilly,** and **not very thirsty.** Children want to be covered, they may moan with the aching muscles, and they are decidedly sluggish and tired. The most characteristic symptom of *Gelsemium* is the **lethargy.** Children may seem like limp noodles, draping themselves over a parent's shoulder, or lying limp in someone's arms. Their eyelids seem heavy and they are sleepy, lacking the energy to even develop a lusty cry. *Gelsemium* is by far the most commonly indicated medicine in children's flu symptoms.

Arsenicum is indicated when the flu begins with digestive disturbance. Children may wake up in the middle of the night and begin the illness with **vomiting.** They soon also develop **diarrhea.** In general, if the first symptom is vomiting, give *Arsenicum*. Children who need this medicine may also be **anxious, chilly,** and **thirsty** for small sips of water. These symptoms may confirm the accuracy of the *Arsenicum* prescription, but it is not necessary for children to fit this classic *Arsenicum* picture to begin using this medicine at the onset of a flu with digestive symptoms.

SECOND STAGE OF FLU

Usually the later stage of the flu in children is characterized by **nasal congestion, headache,** and **cough.** *Bryonia* is the most commonly indicated medicine. Children who need *Bryonia* have a headache and body aches that are decidedly **worse from moving.** They want to lie down and remain still, complaining more if they are moved. They are **thirsty** and **warm.** These children want to be uncovered and complain more if the room is warm. They want windows open and fresh air. They are **irritable** and older children want to be left alone. They soon develop congestion and a **dry cough,** which may be painful because their muscle aches are worse from moving.

If respiratory congestion is the primary symptom, change the medicine to *Pulsatilla* or *Kali-bichromicum.*

The *Pulsatilla* stage has clear or thicker yellow mucus from the nose. The eyes may have some discharge as well. The child wants to move, feels **better from motion** or being carried and rocked. Children who need *Pulsatilla* are **warm, thirstless,** and **clingy.** They want to be held, they cry or whine easily, and seem very dependent. They do not want to be left alone.

Kali-bichromicum is indicated when the nasal discharge or the mucus produced when coughing is **thick** and **green.** These children may have a loose cough, sinus pressure, and night waking from the cough and congestion.

Croup is a fairly common complication of flu in children. Croup is characterized by high-pitched breathing and a barking cough like a seal. The characteristic symptoms are caused by swelling of the throat and larynx. If symptoms occur suddenly in the night with difficult breathing and fear, give *Aconitum* and take your child into the bathroom with the hot shower running. The steam will usually relieve the alarming symptoms. If the barking cough persists, give *Hepar-sulphur*. If the cough later turns loose, with some rattling breathing and hoarseness, switch the medicine to *Spongia-tosta*.

When **diarrhea** persists as a predominant symptom of the flu in children, the three most commonly indicated medicines are *Podophyllum*, *Mercurius*, and *Veratrum album*.

Podophyllum diarrhea is copious, filling up the diaper and running down the legs. Parents wonder where all of this stool comes from. The stool has a foul, offensive odor. Bowel movements may be gushing, and stools are sometimes frothy.

Mercurius (either *Mercurius-solubilis* or *Mercurius-vivus*) fits diarrhea that burns the skin, causing a rash. The stool is watery, and it may be greenish and contain mucus like raw egg whites, or it may be streaked with blood. All of these stool characteristics indicate a very inflamed intestinal tract. *Mercurius* stools are always offensive and acrid, causing redness and pain around the anus. Children who need *Mercurius* are often sweaty and chilly, though they may also feel hot at other times.

Veratrum symptoms tend to be even more severe. Children are cold and shivering, with cold sweats. They also have a nearly unquenchable thirst for cold drinks. The diarrhea is exhausting and painful with abdominal cramping, and these children look quite sick and lethargic.

Acupressure massage

Repeat each maneuver 100 or more times.

TO REDUCE FEVER FROM A FLU OR COLD

Massage the ring finger on the palm side from the base to the tip in one direction only.

Massage along a line in the center of the inside of the forearm from the wrist to the elbow in one direction only.

Massage along a line on the medial anterior surface of the forearm (the pinkie side) from the elbow to the wrist in one direction only.

Rub the temples in the depression at the lateral end (the outer side) of the eyebrows.

Massage the two points at the back of the neck in the hollows on either side of the bony prominence at the base of the skull.

FIRST STAGES OF CONGESTION
(WITH WATERY NASAL DISCHARGE)

Massage the ring finger on the palm side from the tip to the base in one direction only.

Massage along a line on the thumb side of the forearm from the wrist to the elbow in one direction only.

Press on a point at the soft junction of the thumb and index finger.

LATER STAGES OF CONGESTION
(THICK GREEN DISCHARGE)

Massage the ring finger on the palm side from the base to the tip in one direction only.

Massage along a line in the center of the inside of the forearm from the wrist to the elbow in one direction only.

If accompanied by sinus headache, massage the temples and press on the point at the soft junction of the thumb and index finger.

COUGH

Rub the line on the lateral anterior surface of the forearm (the thumb side) from the wrist to the elbow in one direction only.

Massage a point on the center of the chest between the

nipples. Rub outward with both thumbs from the center of the chest to the nipples.

Massage the points on both sides of the back midway between the spine and the edge of the shoulder blades.

Herbs

Echinacea: Non-alcoholic, glycerin preparations of the herb echinacea are prepared specifically for children. Some of them also contain vitamin C. Mix the echinacea with juice or water. Most health food stores stock echinacea preparations. Avoid products that contain other herbs or fillers. Echinacea stimulates the body to produce more white blood cells that fight invasion by viruses or bacteria. Echinacea is not appropriate for allergic symptoms, and should not be used over an extended period of time. Stop when the flu symptoms improve, or after five days.

Directions: Mix with juice or give it straight.

Dosage: For babies under 1 year, 10 drops three times per day; for children over 1 year, 20 drops three times per day.

Windbreaker (from Chinese Modular Solutions): This is a Chinese herbal formula designed for children and available only through health care practitioners. *Yin chao* **Junior**

(from Health Concerns) is a comparable formula. It stimulates a healing reaction in the body, dispels invasion of cold, and relieves mucus production and congestion. Use it at the onset of flu symptoms and continue as long as congestion persists. Shake the bottle before each use. This formula contains alcohol.

Directions: Mix the drops in a small amount of steaming hot water to evaporate the alcohol, then mix this solution with juice.

Dosage: For babies under 1 year, 10 drops three times per day; for children over 1 year, 20 drops three times per day.

Vitamin C

Give babies 500 mg vitamin C in powder form, children 1 to 3 years old 1,000 mg in powder or chewable tablets, and children older than 3 years 1,000 mg twice per day.

Part IV

Adults and Seniors
Adults
Prevention

Maintain a healthy immune system. Many forms of supplements will fortify immunity so that an attack by viruses will be less successful. If you tend to get acute illnesses easily, then begin a program of immune strengthening. See a practitioner (the different types of medical practice are described in Part II) and begin taking supplements on your own. An acupuncturist can advise you about an immune-enhancing herbal formula that will build the strength of your system. These formulas are usually built around astragalus, a potent herb for augmenting the body's protective defenses and stabilizing the exterior against invasion by pathogens and physical stresses such as Cold and Wind. Other supplements have similar immune-enhancing properties.

Several species of mushrooms have significant immune-stimulating effects. Each contains high percentages of

ɪccharides, long-chain sugar molecules that regu-
ɪaɪe ɪmmunity. They activate white blood cells and stimulate antibody production. These mushrooms include
reishi (ganoderma), maitake (grifola), shiitake (lentinus),
polyporus, and tremella. Many preparations of mush-
room combinations in tablet, powder, or liquid extract
form are available at major health food stores and online.

Bovine colostrum has the ability to provide antibodies
directly and stimulate immune function with its potent
combination of lactoferrin that prevents bacteria from
reproducing, lysozyme that destroys pathogenic organ-
isms, and cytokines that stimulate immunoglobulin production. Colostrum is a superfood that should keep your
immune system in peak condition. Take one teaspoon or
two capsules twice a day through the winter months.

Vitamin C at 2–4 grams per day prevents inflammation
and maintains the body's vigilance against infection. Vitamin A is essential to immune function and mucous membrane integrity (see page 64). Take a supplement of 10,000–
25,000 IU of vitamin A derived from fish oil that also
includes vitamin D (400 IU). Zinc has potent immune protective effects. Take 25 mg zinc per day, but if you continue
zinc for an extended period of time you will also need to
take copper to prevent a deficiency (ten-to-one ratio of zinc
to copper). Get a supplement that contains both.

IMMUNE SUPPLEMENTS FOR ADULTS

Mushrooms (reishi, maitake, shiitake)

Colostrum—4 capsules

Vitamin C—2-4 grams

Vitamin A—10,000-25,000 IU with 400 IU vitamin D

Zinc—25 mg with 2 mg copper

Influenzinum is a specific preventive for the flu. You can begin taking *Influenzinum* (9C, 12C, or 30C) if you are exposed to the flu. Take one dose each week for four weeks at that time, or you can take it once a week for four doses during the flu season.

The flu, like other respiratory viruses, spreads from human to human by means of tiny drops of flu-laden fluids. You can minimize your exposure by not shaking hands. Frequent hand washing will also prevent you from inadvertently introducing viruses into your nose and eyes. Avoid touching your nose, mouth, and eyes during flu season to reduce your exposure. Of course, as common courtesy, everyone should cover their mouth when they cough or sneeze to prevent transmission of viruses.

Get plenty of sleep, and eat well. Focus on warm foods during the winter. Soups and stews are excellent sources of concentrated nutrients. Exercise regularly, despite the cold weather. Resist the temptation to go home and lie down after work. Exercise instead. Schedule times for exercise and follow through with your plan. Eat plenty of fruits and vegetables for their vitamin and antioxidant content. Stay warm and avoid getting chilled.

Treatment

Immediately when you begin feeling a scratchy throat or fever, begin a program of vitamin C, echinacea, vitamin A, and a *Yin Chiao* (or similar) formula (see pages 43–45 on the Oriental medicines that help beat the flu). Begin taking *Oscillococcinum* at the onset of symptoms, then switch to the appropriate homeopathic medicine once your symptoms begin to develop clear characteristics. Another effective herb for relieving flu symptoms is black elderberry extract (Sambucol).

Often the initial treatment protocol will stop the illness and the symptoms will go away. If flu symptoms continue, move on to the next phase of treatment. If you have access to an acupuncturist, herbalist, or homeopathic practitioner, seek out their advice. For a discussion of the Chinese herbal approach to flu, see page 42.

You can also choose a homeopathic medicine yourself

FIRST-STAGE TREATMENT FOR FLU (DAY ONE)

	Dosage
Oscillococcinum 200C	½ vial 3 times per day
Vitamin C	4–6 grams per day
Vitamin A	10,000–25,000 IU per day
Yin Chiao	3 times per day
Echinacea	900 mg powder per day, or 3 droppers 3 times per day
Sambucol	2 teaspoons per day

that is indicated for the particular symptoms of your flu. Once specific characteristic symptoms have established themselves, it is possible to find the correct homeopathic medicine. You can also log on to www.cure-guide.com and discover the homeopathic epidemic flu medicine that professional homeopaths have found useful in the current flu epidemic in your part of the country.

The two most frequently indicated homeopathic flu medicines over the past 100 years have been *Gelsemium* and *Bryonia*. Significant differences in the symptom pictures of these two medicines make it easy to decide which is the better fit. They are not the only medicines used to treat the flu, but between them they will probably fit the

CONTRASTING *GELSEMIUM* AND *BRYONIA*

Gelsemium	*Bryonia*
Chilly, with chills down spine	Warm, with desire for cool air
Thirstless	Thirsty
Dull, sleepy, heavy	Dull, but irritable, worried
Worse from movement	All symptoms worse from movement, but restless
Headache at back of head, stiff neck	Headache in forehead, better from pressure, worse with motion

majority of cases.

Bryonia and *Gelsemium* type flus both come on slowly over a six- to twelve-hour period. You begin to feel gradually worse over that time. By the second day you have aching muscles, feel pretty bad, and usually have a headache. A *Bryonia* patient has more pain in the front of the head, which is definitely made worse by moving the head or moving the eyes, and feels better from pressing the hand on the head. A *Gelsemium* patient has pain in the back of the head with stiffness and aching in the neck and across the shoulders. With a *Gelsemium* flu you will not want to move much either, and you may feel worse from moving around, but you avoid movement primarily because you are so tired. The characteristic state of *Gelsemium* is lethargy and fatigue. By contrast, those sufferers who need *Bryonia* will be tired but also restless. *Bryonia* discomfort is worse from motion, but at the same time you feel the urge to move about restlessly in the bed. No position seems comfortable. *Bryonia* patients are thirsty, *Gelsemium* are not. In fact, those who need *Bryonia* are generally warmer and drier, with a desire for air and cool temperatures to calm the heat. *Gelsemium* patients are chilly and sensitive to cold; cold shivers go down their spine. At the same time those who need *Gelsemium* are clammy with the fever, and feelings of heat and cold may alternate. *Bryonia* patients have more coughing and chest symptoms, with a painful cough that aggravates the sore throat. The *Bryonia* cough will also cause chest pains, with the inevitable reaction of pressing the palm to the chest to minimize the movement caused by coughing.

Gelsemium patients do not have the energy to be emotional. *Bryonia* patients are irritable, worried, and fretful. They want to be left alone. *Gelsemium* cases are too exhausted to complain.

BRYONIA—DRY AND ALONE

Brian had to get that report to the marketing department today, headache or no headache. Drink lots of fluids, his wife told the kids when they felt some bug coming on. He stopped at the water cooler in the corridor, noticed he was surprisingly thirsty. Maybe she was right. Flushed, warm, and a little woozy—the signs of flu were unmistakable.

He skipped lunch and slumped over his desk. Made it through a meeting, but now he felt that heavy-headed lethargy he remembered from a similar illness a few years ago. Got to finish the details on this last deal, then I'm out of here, he thought. By 2:30 he knew he better get himself home.

He called home from the car, but Jill was already picking up the kids. No reason to bother her then. He would just get home, make some tea, and relax. Maybe this would pass.

He slept from late afternoon until the next morning. Jill was worried. He told her, "I'm fine, just the flu," and rejected her solicitous care. "Just bring me some water," he said, "and turn down the heat, and keep those kids quiet." Every movement of his head caused the beating there to increase. "You feel hot," she said. When he finally agreed to let Jill take his temperature, it read 102. More Advil.

"I've got to call the office," he said at eight the next morning. "That deal is about to close today."

Then the cough began—dry, racking, and peculiarly painful. Every time he coughed his head hurt more, and that stitching pain in his right side made him wince. His dry mouth, the unquenchable thirst, and the feeling of heat that pervaded his body all attested to the presence of a persistent fever.

Despite feeling truly awful, he wanted to be left alone. Like a dying animal, he became easily irritated if anyone came near him, and his family soon learned to stay away. Luckily, their neighbor was a physician who came over that evening after Jill's anxious call.

"It's not pneumonia," said Dr. Malcolm. "But I do suspect pleurisy, an inflammation of one spot in the lining of the lung. That's why it hurts. I can prescribe some antibiotics, which may help, but I'd suggest you try this first." He left a small vial of white pills labeled Bryonia alba 200. *Brian never needed the antibiotics.*

A third homeopathic medicine for treatment of the flu is *Rhus toxicodendron*. The *Rhus toxicodendron* flu immediately distinguishes itself by extreme restlessness. With all of their aching pains, *Rhus tox* patients feel better from

CONTRASTING *GELSEMIUM* AND *RHUS TOXICODENDRON*

Gelsemium	*Rhus tox*
Chilly, with chills down spine	Chilly, and better from heat
Thirstless	Thirstless
Dull, sleepy, heavy	Extremely restless, cannot get comfortable, anxious
Worse from movement	Better from movement

moving. Constant motion, changing positions, and stretching provide your only relief. If you lie still with a *Rhus tox* flu you begin to ache, which forces you to move. Nighttime is the worst for *Rhus tox* flu patients because of the difficulty remaining in one position. You will toss and turn, looking for relief. Mentally, those who need *Rhus tox* are anxious with a restless mind, and highly emotional—a sudden depression with crying is common. Like *Gelsemium*, *Rhus tox* characteristics include chilliness and sweating. *Rhus tox* patients are also sensitive to cold and feel better from warmth. The headache of both *Rhus tox* and *Gelsemium* has its focus in the back of the neck and head with aching across the shoulders. Those who need *Rhus tox* have a very dry mouth, but despite the dryness are not very thirsty.

Baptisia is another homeopathic medicine that might be indicated by specific characteristics. You would be experiencing a bad flu that comes on quickly with a high fever. Suddenly with a *Baptisia* flu you are very sick and going downhill fast. Mentally, *Baptisia* patients are confused, stupidly dull, and even delirious, sleepy all the time, and unable to even answer questions. The main characteristic is an offensive odor from the sweat, the mouth, and the stool, and *Baptisia* flus are accompanied by both diarrhea and vomiting. The tongue is coated yellow or brown, the throat intensely red, ulcers appear in the mouth, and the gums ooze blood.

Seniors
Prevention

The special flu risk for older people is not their age, but the presence of other underlying disease states, weakened immunity, and poor nutritional status that makes them more susceptible to the complications of flu. It is essential that seniors take the immune system supplements outlined in this chapter for adults during the fall and winter months.

The human body was not designed to last seventy or

eighty years. Prior to the twentieth century, the lifespan of humans was about sixty years—if they made it to age forty. The body needs support to maintain a state of health and resilience past sixty. Seniors need to take antioxidants on a daily basis in the form of vitamin C (1,000 mg), vitamin E (400 IU), CoQ10 (100 mg), and selenium (200 mcg). Taking fish oil and getting adequate amounts of vitamins A and D are essential steps to maintain the health of joints and mucous membranes. Cod liver oil contains both the valuable omega-3 fats of fish and vitamins A and D. Most seniors also benefit from taking digestive enzymes that assist in the absorption of nutrients, since the body's production of these enzymes decreases with age.

In addition to supplements, the best preventive for seniors is to manage any chronic disease process with supportive therapies. Whether you have diabetes, heart disease, high blood pressure, or an inflammatory condition like arthritis, specific treatment with alternative healing systems can restore a healthy balance in the body and develop an optimal level of health. This can reduce the need for medications such as painkillers, and prevent any worsening of disorders that might call for more drugs.

The perspective of Oriental medicine provides important therapeutic benefits for seniors. Most seniors have a fundamental energetic deficiency. Simply put, as people age, the body's store of energy and vitality begins to run low. Oriental medicine practitioners can diagnose the specific forms of energetic deficiency present in any individual, but unless the patient takes measures to build energy, the deficiency will worsen. There are many Chinese herbal formulas that "tonify," or increase the body's energetic foundation. Most of these formulas are built around the herbs ginseng, astragalus, rehmannia, and angelica. All manufacturers of Oriental medicine formulas provide a variety of choices to build energy, strengthen immune function, and prepare seniors for a winter season that threatens their health. The flexibility of Chinese herbal formulas allows for individuality and selectivity in applying the appropriate balance of herbs to correct the wide variety of deficiency states that aging produces. A licensed practitioner of Oriental medicine or acupuncture can advise you about the specific formulas that will benefit your individual health and state of balance.

If you get sick with the flu or other respiratory illness, you should stop herbal tonification formulas, especially if they contain ginseng. Also stop taking any vitamin supplement that contains ginseng. Tonification formulas can drive disease deeper into the body. After a complete recovery, you can begin them again. During an illness, you should replace the tonification formula with herbs specific to the disease state that has temporarily gained dominance in your body.

Many foods and supplements also have the ability to build the body's store of energy and thereby strengthen immunity. Royal jelly is one of the most profound of these foods. Prepared for the queen bee in a hive by worker bees, this food is one of the most concentrated tonifying substances known. It builds reproductive energy in the queen bee, and in humans it produces fundamental energy or *Qi*, the fuel source that propels the immune system. Use the pure form of royal jelly that comes packaged in small tubs at your health food store. The usual dose is one-quarter teaspoon per day, preferably taken in the morning.

Treatment for pneumonia

At the first signs of the flu, seniors need to immediately begin bolstering the immune system response and stabilizing cells to prevent the damage that results from accumulation of fluids in the lungs and airways. Vitamin C, Sambucol, *Yin Chiao*, echinacea, and *Oscillococcinum* can all be started at the onset of the flu. Seniors should keep these on hand during the winter months to begin at the first signs of flu-like illness. All can be purchased at any large health food store or online. The discussion of homeopathic medicines (page 91–97) and Chinese herbs (pages 42–46) for adults applies equally to seniors.

Pneumonia is the major complication of the flu for seniors and the primary reason that fatalities occur in flu illnesses. An estimated 90 percent of influenza deaths occur in people over 65 years old (Thompson, 2003). Pneumonia can be caused by the flu virus or it can occur as a secondary bacterial infection. A bacterial pneumonia typically occurs after the flu symptoms fade. You recover from the flu and then get sick again with a fever, shortness of breath, chest pain, and cough. This secondary infection is a sign of a weakened immune system and it needs to be treated vigorously.

Seniors who have pneumonia must take antibiotics. This is a life-threatening illness. However, antibiotics have limitations. If your pneumonia is viral (caused by the flu virus directly), antibiotics will do no good. They may prevent secondary bacterial infections, but they will not improve the pneumonia. The failure of antibiotics and the inability of conventional medicine to treat viral pneumonias represent a major contributing cause of flu deaths in seniors. The second problem with antibiotics is bacterial resistance. Many strains of bacteria responsible for pneumonia are simply resistant to the effects of antibiotics. The antibiotic resistance rate for pneumococcal respiratory disease has steadily increased since at least 1998, when a resistance tracking surveillance program began keeping records. For example, during the period 1998 through 2002, resistance to penicillin of *Streptococcus pneumoniae* from lower respiratory tract sites increased from 14.7 to 18.4 percent, and resistance to the antibiotic azythromycin increased from 22.7 to 27.5 percent (Karlowsky, 2003).

Two forms of treatment have a long history of curing pneumonia—homeopathy and Chinese herbal medicine. Before the era of antibiotics, both of these systems produced sophisticated treatment regimens for pneumonia. The treatment of pneumonia with homeopathic medicines or Chinese herbal formulas, in addition to antibiotics and hospital care, will reduce the incidence of unnecessary deaths. Pneumonia is not the realm for home prescribing. An experienced practitioner needs to supervise the care of patients with pneumonia. The following guidelines are illustrative of the sophistication of these alternative medical systems and their ability to manage serious complications of the flu alongside conventional medical interventions. In integrative practices, where the best of conventional and holistic medical models co-exist, pneumonia cases will fare much better and mortality will decrease.

HOMEOPATHY

Homeopaths generally distinguish between possible prescriptions on the basis of individual symptoms. This is true for both flu and pneumonia. When considering pneumonia, homeopaths also separate the possible medicines into groups that correspond to the worsening stages of the disease. Dr. Douglas Borland defined these pneumonia stages (Borland, 1940):

1. An incipient stage of onset during the first twenty-four hours of illness
2. Developed pneumonia, after the first twenty-four hours
3. Complicated pneumonia, when pathogens have invaded deep levels of the body and bloodstream (it is said to be septic) and the person is feeling very ill
4. Creeping pneumonia, with infection spreading to different areas of the lungs and bronchi
5. Lingering pneumonia, with severe symptoms that continue long after the initial siege of the acute disease state, with persistent cough, severe chest pain, blue-colored skin, and heart failure

These different stages call for different classes of medicines, beginning with superficial fever treatment for the first flash of illness in stage one. Once the characteristic signs of pneumonia appear (high fever, evidence of fluid in the lungs, deep cough, and weakness), a set of deeper-acting medicines is appropriate. If symptoms worsen, a third group of medicines enters into consideration—medicines associated with toxic, septic conditions that correspond to gravely ill people who will undoubtedly be hospitalized. The fourth stage features spreading pneumonia, with the patient gradually worsening and sites of localized infection progressing. These patients are quite ill and obviously failing; the medicines that correspond to this stage are typical for dispersed localized infections in the chest. The fifth group consists of patients who are simply not improving over an extended period, becoming weaker and in serious danger of succumbing to the infection. One of the medicines of this fifth group, *Carbo vegetabilis,* is actually known for its ability to seemingly revive the dead. The lungs are filling with fluid, the face is becoming bluish-purple from lack of oxygen, and the heart is failing. The fact that homeopathy was able to rescue some of these patients in the era preceding the advent of antibiotics attests to the power of these medicines.

ORIENTAL MEDICINE

Traditional Chinese medicine views pneumonia as a later

HOMEOPATHIC MEDICINES FOR PNEUMONIA (BORLAND)

Incipient stage	*Aconite, Belladonna, Ferrum phosphoricum, Ipecac*
Developed pneumonia	*Bryonia, Phosphorus, Veratrum viride, Chelidonium*
Complicated pneumonia	*Baptisia, Mercurius, Rhus toxicodendron, Pyrogen, Hepar sulphuris, Lachesis*
Creeping pneumonia	*Pulsatilla, Natrum sulphuricum, Senega, Lobelia*
Lingering pneumonia	*Antimony tartaricum, Carbo vegetabilis, Kali carbonicum, Arsenicum, Lycopodium, Sulphur*

stage in the progression from an exterior condition to an interior condition. The attack by External Wind or External Wind Heat penetrates the superficial level of Defensive *Qi*, resulting in typical flu symptoms. If the disease progresses deeper to an internal *Qi* level, the resulting condition is pneumonia, or Internal Lung Heat.

Internal Lung Heat may be dry or contain phlegm (Lung Phlegm-Heat). Either of these two conditions can be treated with Chinese herbal formulas and acupuncture. Usually

ACUTE ILLNESS WITH COUGH

External Wind ————————————→ Internal Heat

The traditional Chinese medicine view of the progression of cough symptoms from the attack of External Wind stage to the pneumonia stage of Internal Lung Heat.

there is considerable congestion in the chest with pneumonia in seniors, so practitioners will prescribe Lung Phlegm-Heat formulas that contain herbs such as scutellaria or coptis to clear Lung Heat, plus trichosanthis, arisaematis, fritillary, and pinellia to clear Phlegm. The formulas and herbal combinations will clear Heat and Phlegm, and move *Qi* in the chest, to break up the congestion that underlies pneumonia. Acupuncture points are also used that clear Phlegm and Heat from the lungs and restore the downward movement of lung *Qi*. For example, points on the Lung channel are used to treat cough and pneumonia (LU 1,5,6). Large Intestine 11 clears Heat, Conception Vessel 12 in the center of the chest disperses *Qi* and expands the chest, Stomach 40 disperses Phlegm, and Triple Burner points 5,6 spread the *Qi* and relieve Heat.

Conclusion

The dangers of the flu and the probability of another worldwide flu pandemic make flu treatment an important public health policy issue. The only hope for reducing the number of fatalities from the flu depends on applying an integrative medicine approach. Epidemiologists and public health organizations represent the first line of defense against the flu. They have the responsibility for identifying viruses, isolating cases of bird flu victims, and quarantining and destroying flocks of birds that transmit viruses. Hospital and emergency medical services need contingency plans for coping with the requirements of a widespread epidemic in all major population centers around the world.

Once a virus has spread into the human population, integrative medical approaches that include homeopathy, herbal medicine, and nutritional supplements offer the most effective program for flu treatment. If your health care system does not include these modalities, then you should have them in place for your own family's health care plan.

Prepare for this year's flu with a home cold and flu kit. Collect the supplies you will need and your family will be ready for the onset of those viruses that pass from one family member to another.

ADULT FLU KIT

Have on hand a packet or bottle of each of the following. If anybody has been exposed to the flu, or is showing early signs of the flu, you will need to start right away with this reinforcement program for your immune defenses.

Influenzinum 30C or *Dolivaxil* 9C for prevention

Oscillococcinum 200 at the first signs of symptoms

Vitamin C—powder or capsules, 1,000 mg

Vitamin A&D—capsules, 10,000 IU vitamin A with 400 IU vitamin D

Yin Chiao—liquid extract or pills

Echinacea—liquid extract

Sambucol—liquid extract/syrup

Homeopathic medicines:
  Bryonia 30C
  Gelsemium 30C

CHILDREN'S FLU KIT

In addition to the adult flu kit, keep a bottle of each of the following items on hand for children under 12.

Vitamin C—chewable tablets, 500 mg

Windbreaker—from Chinese Modular Solutions (Rx only) or

Yin Chiao Junior—from Health Concerns (Rx only)

Homeopathic medicines:
> *Belladonna* 30C
> *Arsenicum* 30C
> *Pulsatilla* 30C

References

Barak, V, *et al.* The effect of herbal remedies on the production of human inflammatory and anti-inflammatory cytokines. *Israel Medical Association Journal* 2002 Nov.; 4(11 Suppl):944–946.

Belshe, RB, *et al.* Serum antibody responses after intradermal vaccination against influenza. *New England Journal of Medicine* 2004 Nov. 25; 351(22).

Bodinet, C, *et al.* Host-resistance increasing activity of root extracts from Echinacea species. *Planta Medica* 1993; 59(Suppl): A672.

Borland, DM. Pneumonias: Postgraduate lectures delivered at the London Homoeopathic Hospital, Spring 1939. *Homoeopathy* 1940 (reprinted as a series of articles).

Burger, RA, *et al.* Echinacea-induced cytokine production by human macrophages. *International Journal Immunopharmacology* 1997 July; 19(7):371–379.

CDC. Prevention and control of influenza: Recommendations of the Advisory Committee on Immunization Practices (ACIP). *MMWR* 2001; 50(RR04):1–46.

CDC. Preliminary assessment of the effectiveness of the 2003–2004 inactivated influenza vaccine—Colorado, December 2003. *MMWR* 2004 Jan 16; 53(01):8–11.

CDC. Deaths: Final Data for 2002. *National Vital Statistics Reports* 2004(a) Oct. 12; 53(5).

Chandra, RK. Immunological aspects of human milk. *Nutrition Review* 1978; 36:265.

Cooper, NJ, *et al.* Effectiveness of neuraminidase inhibitors in treatment and prevention of influenza A and B: systematic review and meta-analyses of randomised controlled trials. *British Medical Journal* 2003 June 7; 326(7401):1235.

Coulamy, A. Survey of the prescription habits of homeopathic doctors on the subject of a single medication: Influenzinum. *French Society of Homeopathy Conference Notes: The Prescription in Homeopathy* 1998:1–16.

Davies, JR and Grilli, EA. Natural or vaccine-induced antibody as a predictor of immunity in the face of natural challenge with influenza viruses. *Epidemiology and Infection* 1989 Aug.; 103(1):217.

Ferley, JP, *et al.* A controlled evaluation of a homoeopathic preparation in the treatment of influenza-like syndromes. *British Journal of Clinical Pharmacology* 1989; 27:329–335.

Fratkin, J. *Chinese Herbal Patent Medicines*. Boulder, Colo.: Shya Publications, 2001.

Gamblin, SJ, *et al.* The structure and receptor binding properties of the 1918 influenza hemagglutinin. *Sci-

ence 2004 March 19; 303(5665):1838–1842.

Goldman, AS, *et al.* Immunologic factors in human milk during the first year of lactation. *Journal of Pediatrics* 1982; 100:563.

Hanson, LA. Breastfeeding provides passive and likely long-lasting active immunity. *Annals of Allergy Asthma and Immunology* 1998 Dec.; 81(6):523–533.

Izurieta HS, *et al.* Influenza and the rates of hospitalization for respiratory disease among infants and young children. *New England Journal of Medicine* 2000 Jan. 27; 342(4):232–239.

Karlowsky, JA, *et al.* Factors associated with relative rates of antimicrobial resistance among Streptococcus pneumoniae in the United States: results from the TRUST surveillance program (1998–2002). *Clinical Infectious Diseases* 2003 April 15; 36:963–970.

Kenney, RT, *et al.* Dose sparing with intradermal injection of influenza vaccine. *New England Journal of Medicine* 2004 Nov. 25; 351(22).

Lasky T, *et al.* Guillain-Barré syndrome and the 1992–1993 and 1993–1994 influenza vaccines. *New England Journal of Medicine* 1998; 339:1797–1802.

Li, KS, *et al.* Genesis of a highly pathogenic and potentially pandemic H5N1 influenza virus in eastern Asia. *Nature* 2004; 430:209–213.

Lindenmuth, GF and Lindenmuth, EB. The efficacy of Echinacea compound herbal tea preparation on the severity and duration of upper respiratory and flu symptoms: a randomized, double-blind placebo-controlled study. *Journal Alternative and Complementary Medicine* 2000 Aug; 6(4):327–334.

Maeda, T, *et al*. Failure of inactivated influenza A vaccine to protect healthy children aged 6–24 months. *Pediatrics International* 2004; 46:122–125.

Marks, JS and Halpin, TJ. Guillain-Barré syndrome in recipients of A/New Jersey influenza vaccine. *Journal American Medical Association* 1980; 243(42):2490–2494.

Melchart, D, *et al*. Results of five randomized studies on the immunomodulatory activity of preparations of Echinacea. *Journal Alternative and Complementary Medicine* 1995; 1:145–160.

Neuzil, KM, *et al*. The effect of influenza on hospitalizations, outpatient visits, and courses of antibiotics in children. *New England Journal of Medicine* 2000 Jan. 27; 342(4):225–231.

Oddy, WH, *et al*. The relation of breastfeeding and body mass index to asthma and atopy in children: a prospective cohort study to age 6 years. *American Journal Public Health* 2004 Sept.; 94(9):1531–1537.

Papp, R, *et al.* Oscillococcinum in patients with influenza-like syndromes: a placebo-controlled double-blind evaluation. *British Homeopathic Journal* 1998; 87:69–76.

Pawelec, G, *et al.* Pathways to a robust immune response in the elderly. *Immunology Allergy Clinics of North America* 2003 Feb; 23(1):1–13.

Perko, SJ. *The Homeopathic Treatment of Influenza: Surviving Influenza Epidemics and Pandemics, Past, Present and Future with Homeopathy.* San Antonio, Texas: Benchmark Homeopathic Publications, 1999.

Reddy, NR and Sathe, SK, eds. *Food Phytates,* Boca Raton, Fla.: CRC Press, 2002.

Safranek, TJ, *et al.* Reassessment of the association between Guillain-Barré syndrome and receipt of swine influenza vaccine in 1976–1977: results of a two-state study. Expert Neurology Group. *American Journal of Epidemiology* 1991; 133(9):940–951.

Sendi, P, *et al.* Intranasal influenza vaccine in a working population. *Clinical Infectious Disease* 2004 April 1; 38(7):974–980.

Steinman, RM and Pope, M. Exploiting dendritic cells to improve vaccine efficacy. *Journal Clinical Investigation* 2002; 109:1519–1526.

Thompson, WW, *et al.* Mortality associated with influenza and respiratory syncytial virus in the United States.

Journal American Medical Association 2003 Jan. 8; 289(2):179–186.

Watkins, BA and Seifert, MF. Food lipids and bone health, in *Food Lipids and Health,* McDonald, RE and Min, EB, eds. New York: Marcel Dekker, Inc., 1996.

Zakay-Rones, Z, *et al.* Inhibition of several strains of influenza virus in vitro and reduction of symptoms by an elderberry extract (Sambucus nigra L.) during an outbreak of influenza B Panama. *Journal Alternative and Complementary Medicine* 1995 Winter; 1(4):361–369.

Zakay-Rones Z, *et al.* Randomized study of the efficacy and safety of oral elderberry extract in the treatment of influenza A and B virus infections. *Journal International Medical Research* 2004 March-April; 32(2):132–140.

Resources

Recommended Books

Everybody's Guide to Homeopathic Medicines by Dana Ullman and Stephen Cummings (JP Tarcher, 1997, 374 pages), and *Homeopathic Medicine for Children & Infants* by Dana Ullman (JP Tarcher, 1992, 256 pages). The classics for quick homeopathic prescribing for acute ailments.

Smart Medicine for a Healthier Child: A Practical A-Z Reference to Natural and Conventional Treatments for Infants and Children by Janet Zand, OMD and Robert Rountree, MD (Avery Publishing Group, 2003, 544 pages). This book contains extended discussions of each symptom or disease in alphabetic order, with corresponding conventional and alternative treatment methods (homeopathy, herbs, and acupressure).

Homeopathic Self-Care: The Quick and Easy Guide for the Whole Family by Robert Ullman and Judyth Reichenberg-Ullman (Prima Publishing, 1997, 433 pages). A homeopathic home prescriber with step-by-step instructions and carefully constructed visual presentations in a graphic format that proceeds logically and simply to guide choices to the correct medicine.

The Homeopathic Emergency Guide by Thomas Kruzel (North Atlantic Books, 1992). This is the best supplementary book for detailed homeopathic descriptions of acute symptoms that will help to differentiate the alternative prescriptions.

The Homeopathic Treatment of Influenza: Surviving Influenza Epidemics and Pandemics, Past, Present and Future with Homeopathy by Sandra J. Perko, PhD (Benchmark Homeopathic Publications, 1999, 382 pages). A detailed history and symptomatology of the flu, including the 1918 pandemic, and an exhaustive homeopathic treatment guide. By far the best homeopathic text on influenza ever written.

The Great Influenza: The Epic Story of the Deadliest Plague in History by John M. Barry (Viking, 2004, 546 pages). A remarkable recounting of the 1918 pandemic and its impact on world history and medical science.

Practitioner referral directories on the Internet

American Association of Naturopathic Physicians
www.naturopathic.org
American Association of Oriental Medicine
www.aaom.org

American Holistic Medical Association
www.holisticmedicine.org
Council for Homeopathic Certification
www.homeopathicdirectory.com
Holistic Pediatric Association
www.hpakids.org
International Chiropractic Pediatric Association
www.icpa4kids.com
National Center for Homeopathy
www.homeopathic.org

Body movement therapies on the Internet

Yoga
www.yogajournal.com
Tai chi
www.thetaichisite.com
Chi gong
www.alternativehealing.org
Aikido
www.aikiweb.com
Alexander technique
www.alexandertechnique.com
Feldenkrais technique
www.feldenkrais.com

Sources of homeopathic medicines and herbs

Homeopathic Educational Service
   www.homeopathic.com
   510-649-0294
Boiron
   www.boiron.com
   800-BLUTUBE
Dolisos
   www.dolisos.com
   800-DOLISOS
Kan Herbs and Chinese Modular Solutions
   www.kanherb.com
   800-543-5233
Crane Herb Company
   www.craneherb.com
   800-227-4118

Visit Dr. Neustaedter's website. Subscribe to his free email newsletter and view the current updates on this year's flu and its treatment. www.cure-guide.com